"Dr. Erik Schott's *LGBTQI Workbook for CBT* aims high, presenting a comprehensive set of exercises and fun activities that are intended to help members of LGBTQI communities build character, develop resilience, and adopt constructive thoughts, feelings, and actions. The workbook can also be recommended for therapists as a resource for increasing fluency in issues relevant to sexual minorities."

—**Vivienne Cass, PhD**, Adjunct Associate Professor (prior),
Curtin University, author of *A Quick Guide to the Cass Theory of
Gay & Lesbian Identity Formation*

"Dr. Schott's *LGBTQI Workbook for CBT* is a practical and most useful resource for social work students and mental health practitioners in the field. The workbook provides a panoply of exercises, resources, and tools for self-reflection, action planning, and strengthening of the therapeutic alliance via the lens of affirming practice and principles of CBT."

—**Michael P. Dentato, PhD, MSW**, Associate Professor of Social
Work, Loyola University Chicago, author of *Social Work Practice
with the LGBTQ Community*

"This is a welcome new addition to the genre of LGBTQI books where few are published anymore. A comprehensive and inclusive guide for queer folks to use cognitive behavioral therapy tools, it is filled with practical and easy exercises to use through handouts and resources. The issues tackled in this book within the LGBTQI community are inclusive in a clever way given the book being a short workbook. I highly recommend it to the queer community and those working with them."

—**Joe Kort, PhD, MSW, MA**, therapist and co-director of
Modern Sex Therapy Institutes (LGBTQIA Affirmative Therapy
certificate), author of *LGBTQ Clients in Therapy*

"*LGBTQI Workbook for CBT* is a very welcomed answer to the perennial question about affirmative practice with queer people: But, how do you do *that*? This text is imminently readable, extremely pragmatic, and perfectly economical in breadth and depth—for both the client system and clinicians alike. Dr. Schott has distilled CBT in an effective way for all users, while simultaneously infusing CBT with the core ethos and practical strategies that promote queer validation and that help users along a path of healing from minority stress and anti-LGBTQ+ oppression. This should not only be part of the intervention toolbox when working with LGBTQ+ people—but it should be part of the educational archive for training practitioners."

—**Tyler M. Argüello, PhD, DCSW, LCSW**, Associate Professor
of Social Work, California State University, Sacramento, author of
Queer Social Work: Cases for LGBTQ+ Affirmative Practice

LGBTQI Workbook For CBT

Cognitive-Behavioral Therapy (CBT) is one of the most popular evidence-based interventions in the world, but little has been done to explore how it affects different groups of people, such as the lesbian, gay, bisexual, transgender, queer, and intersex (LGBTQI) community. The *LGBTQI Workbook for CBT* is filled with hands-on, practical perspectives for readers who are seeking a new point-of-view or for clinicians and students seeking additional tools, competence, and humility when working with sexual and gender minorities.

The workbook focuses on skill building and addresses techniques for personal self-assessment, cognitive and behavioral activation, psychoeducation, and therapist resources. Incorporating structured learning tools to promote professional responsibility as well as ethically driven and evidence-based practices, this text aims to promote empowerment. Applied activities are available in multiple reproducible worksheets and handouts to utilize in session, in the classroom, in the field, and in life.

The *LGBTQI Workbook for CBT* is an invaluable resource for interested members of the LGBTQI community, beginner or experienced clinicians, and students working with sexual and gender minority clients. It is an excellent supplementary text for graduate students in social work, psychology, nursing, psychiatry, professional counseling, marriage and family therapy, and other healing professions such as medicine, acupuncture, or physical therapy.

Dr. Erik Schott is a clinical associate professor at the University of Southern California (USC) and a licensed clinical social worker in Los Angeles. He is a certified Eye Movement Desensitization and Reprocessing (EMDR) psychotherapist; holds specialized training in Emotionally Focused Couples Therapy (EFT) and CBT; and has expertise in LGBTQI social work, childhood neurodevelopmental life issues, HIV/AIDS, diversity, equity, and inclusion (DEI) pedagogy, and instructional design.

LGBTQI Workbook For CBT

Erik Schott

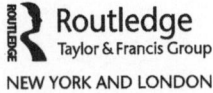
Routledge
Taylor & Francis Group

NEW YORK AND LONDON

First published 2021
by Routledge
605 Third Avenue, New York, NY 10158

and by Routledge
2 Park Square, Milton Park, Abingdon, Oxon, OX14 4RN

Routledge is an imprint of the Taylor & Francis Group, an informa business

Library of Congress Cataloging-in-Publication Data
Names: Schott, Erik, author.
Title: LGBTQI workbook for CBT / Erik Schott.
Description: New York, NY: Routledge Books, 2021. |
Includes bibliographical references and index.
Identifiers: LCCN 2020043271 | ISBN 9780367544362 (hardback) |
ISBN 9780367513788 (paperback) | ISBN 9781003089285 (ebook)
Subjects: LCSH: Sexual minorities—Psychology. |
Sexual minorities—Psychology—Problems, exercises, etc. |
Cognitive therapy—Problems, exercises, etc.
Classification: LCC RC451.4.G39 S36 2021 | DDC 616.89/142500866—dc23
LC record available at https://lccn.loc.gov/2020043271

ISBN: 978-0-367-54436-2 (hbk)
ISBN: 978-0-367-51378-8 (pbk)
ISBN: 978-1-003-08928-5 (ebk)

Typeset in Frutiger
by codeMantra

Dedication

To Michael – go make history!

To the LGBTQI+ community – we need this book until we don't, so keep working at it every day.

To the social workers, psychotherapists, and healing professionals – continue to stay educated and strong for the clients and communities you serve.

In honor of the above, certain proceeds from this workbook will be donated to the following:

The LA LGBT Center, Los Angeles, California

The Center for Transyouth Health and Development at Children's Hospital Los Angeles, California

Casa Um, São Paulo, Brazil

CAMP Rehoboth Community Center, Rehoboth Beach, Delaware

Contents

Part 4: Psychoeducational Handouts and Worksheets   61

Part 5: Therapist Handouts and Worksheets   87

About the Author

Dr. Erik Schott, EdD, MSW, LCSW, is a clinical associate professor at University of Southern California (USC), licensed clinical social worker, educational psychologist, and instructional designer in Los Angeles. The nexus of his clinical practice, teaching, and scholarship profile is a commitment to lesbian, gay, bisexual, queer, and intersex (LGBTQI) social work, child development, attention-deficit/hyperactivity disorder (ADHD), couple therapy, HIV/AIDS, and diversity, equity, and inclusion (DEI) pedagogy. He is a certified Eye Movement Desensitization and Reprocessing (EMDR) psychotherapist and holds specialized training in Emotionally Focused Couples Therapy (EFT) and Cognitive Behavioral Therapy (CBT). He has worked as a front-line clinician and was a program director at the Serra Project, a housing non-profit that organized in response to the outbreak of the HIV/AIDS pandemic – a crisis that rages on and must be ended. At USC, Schott teaches generalist to advanced clinical practice courses and has initiated innovative curriculum design on LGBTQI clinical, policy, and community organizing practice. At the vanguard of online education, Erik created immersive coursework to address social stigma for the LGBTQI community in both North and South America. He co-edited the book *Transformative Social Work Practice* (Sage, 2016). Follow him on Twitter @EriksEasel.

Disclaimer

As we live and learn on these territories, we must keep in mind the community struggles for self-determination and the colonial legacies of scholarly and clinical practices. We recognize and acknowledge that the University of Southern California, the Suzanne Dworak-Peck School of Social Work, and Silver Lake Psychotherapy were formed and grown on the lands stewarded by the Tongva People. For thousands of years, the Tongva people lived on this land we occupy today. We also recognize the Chumash, Tataviam, Serrano, Cahuilla, Juaneno, and Luiseno People for the land that USC occupies around Southern California.

This workbook is a resource to support personal self-growth. It can be a toolkit and can be utilized conjunctively with traditional psychotherapies. It is not a diagnosis tool, nor is it a substitute for the treatment of a mental health or physical disorder or condition. If you are feeling suicidal, please immediately call 911 or your regional emergency contact. You are advised to contact a mental health professional if you are having any difficulties. You can, of course, use this workbook on your own but do so at your own risk. The author and publisher of this workbook are not responsible for the behavior of those who have not followed the above advice. No one workbook can completely cover every issue relating to the LGBTQI community utilizing CBT, and there may be omissions.

This workbook is dedicated to those who want to gain psychological and behavioral insights with an LGBTQI intersectional lens. The compilation addresses techniques for personal self-assessment, cognitive and behavioral activation, psychoeducational tools, and therapist resources. It is a hands-on and practical resource for the novice social work student to the seasoned clinician looking for a new point-of-view with a toolbox attached. It is for human beings who wish to self-reflect and set new personal goals as many of the handouts and worksheets do not necessarily require an LGBTQI identity for them to be relevant exercises. Dr. Schott's creative science-based and artistic application of CBT to the various handouts and worksheets reflects the desire to create an individualized action plan for every person seeking positive change. One schema or belief from this workbook is that, over time, behaviors are learned, for the good, the bad, or even the neutral. The promising news is that, if the effort is applied, we can unlearn old behaviors, replace them with new ones, and keep practicing and growing. Empowerment is the general goal of this workbook. As human beings, some of our "universal" goals on a treatment plan should include proper nutrition, regular exercise, sufficient sleep, maintaining healthy relationships, balancing work-life responsibilities, and attentive self-reflection, along with diligent self-care. This workbook was designed with the consideration of these critical guiding "universal" goals.

Current Life Selfie

In the space below, place a selfie, doodle, drawing, stickers, stamps, words, or cut-and-paste printed images that represent what you feel and think about yourself currently.

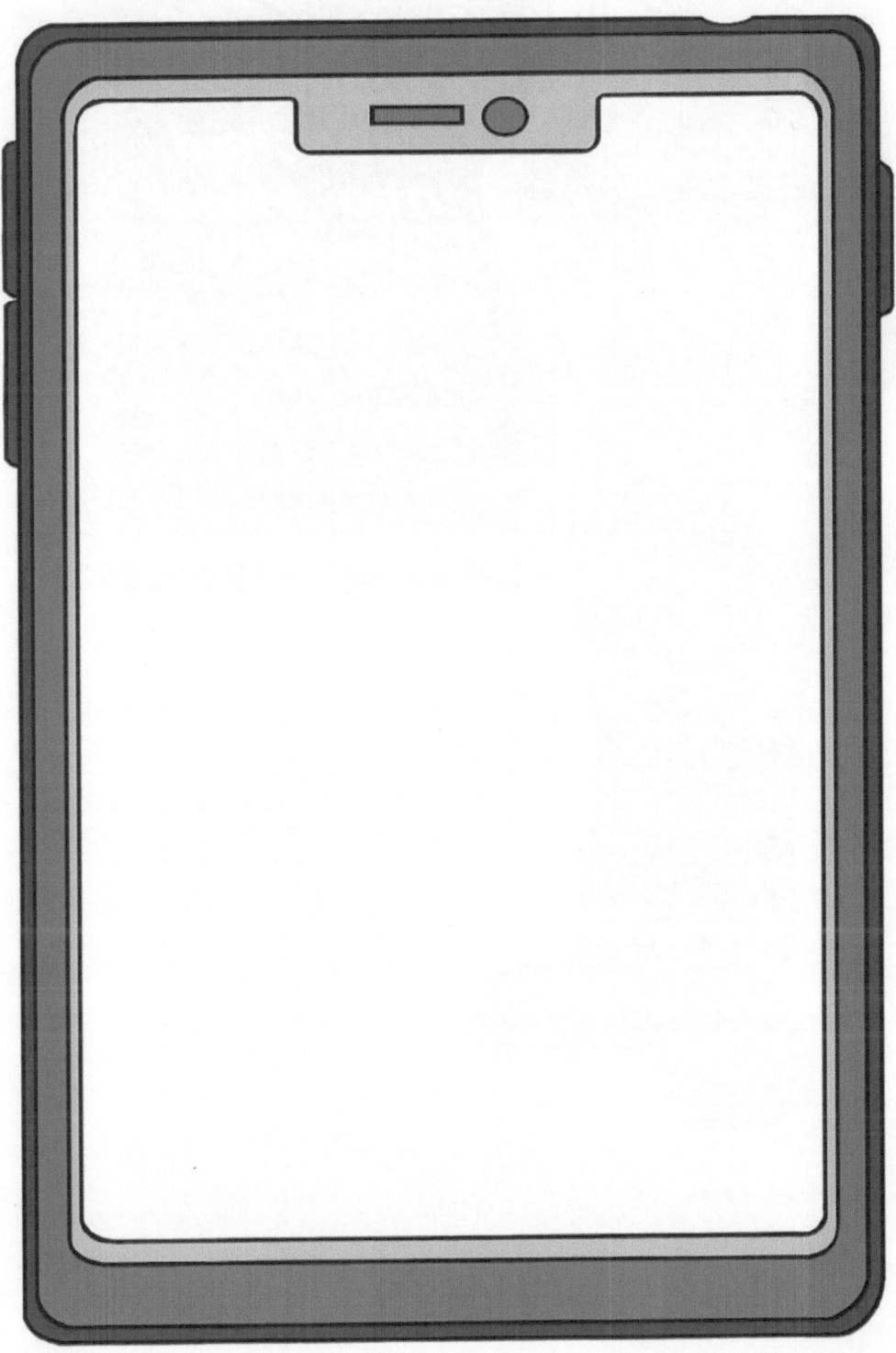

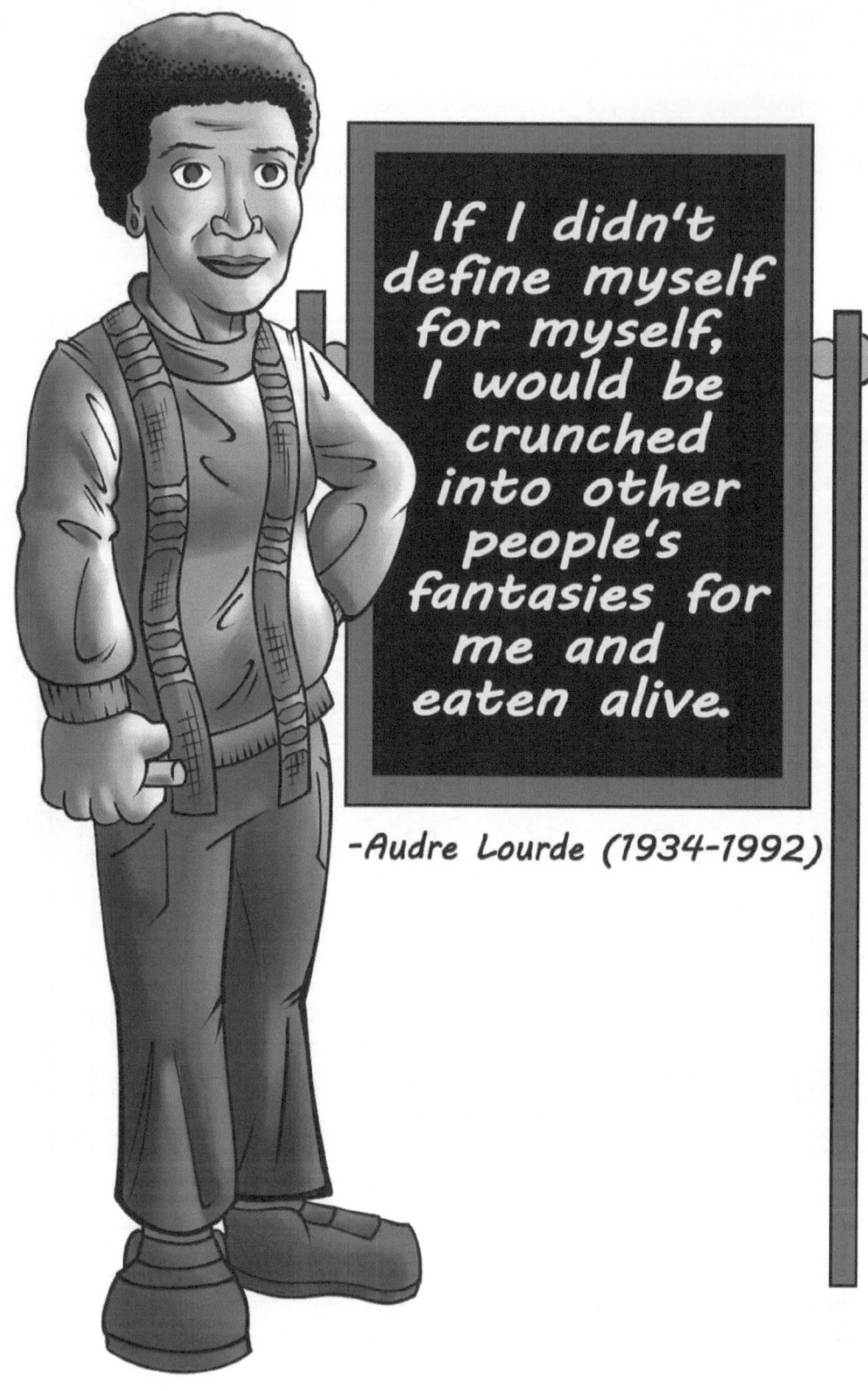

The word *assess* comes from the Latin *assidere*, which means to sit beside. Literally, to assess means to sit beside the learner. Assessment is a conversation. It is an ongoing dialog that is never finished. It is a pivot, a volley, a wedge, or whatever metaphor works for your mind – go with that.

As work for this text began, a dear colleague was overheard, taking a phone call from her anxious daughter. She told them to "go change your location." This powerful directive resonated with me as the goal of this workbook, sometimes literally changing your physical location as a technique, but also learning to change the location of negative thoughts in ones' mind. We have learned everything; it can all be unlearned with consistent motivation and practice. Homework is key to your cognitive and behavioral self-analysis journey.

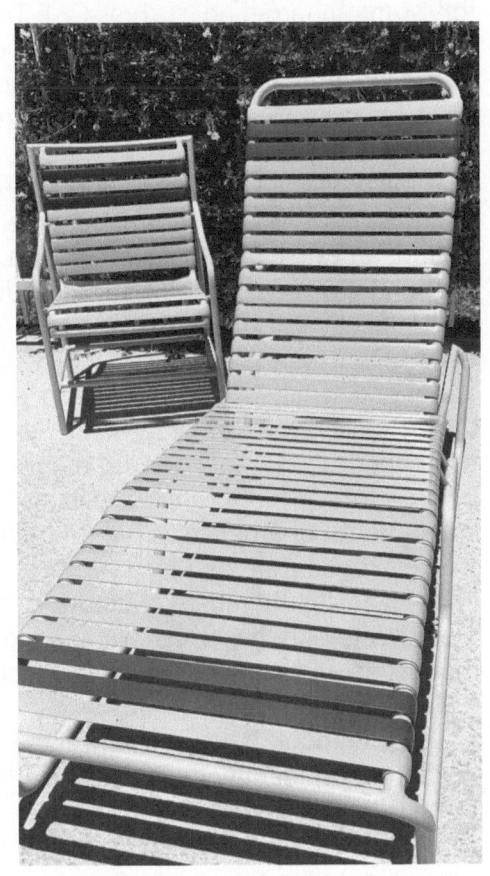

HOW TO USE THIS WORKBOOK

The purpose of this workbook is to help the reader learn enhanced positive coping skills to make life changes and improve quality of life. Cognitive Behavioral Therapy is the umbrella from which the workbook takes its framework. CBT is an evidence-based practice that has advanced the practices of many mental health practitioners. This workbook was designed to facilitate the integration of empirically support therapies like CBT and integrate them into everyday clinical practice and self-reflection, specifically with the LGBTQI community. This workbook was designed to help the individual become more insightful and help them assess their readiness for change. Change requires one to grow, but growth with a structured workbook and the assistance of a mental health therapist can catapult oneself in a new direction emotionally and physically quicker than just working alone.

Research has demonstrated preliminary support for the first interventions adapted to address the LGBTQI community's co-occurring health problems at their source in minority stress. In the translation of science into clinical practice, there is currently great opportunities in helping clinicians translate LGBTQI affirmative treatment guidelines into evidence-based practice. In approaching treatment with clients using an LGBTQI Affirmative Therapy (AT) framework, the therapist is adhering to clinical best practices as there are currently no specific evidence-based interventions (EBI) for LGBTQI populations. Because of this lack of EBIs, therapist must think critically though a trauma-informed lens as to what skills they will focus on in sessions with clients. While the research and clinical guidelines on AT is not always clearly demarcated, the framework can have some positive impact (Pachankis, Hatzenbuehler, Rendina, Safren, & Parsons, 2015).

The AT framework can help build client and therapist rapport, complete LGBTQI sensitive biological-psychological-social assessments, and in choosing interventions for symptom targeting, such as CBT. The role of an AT therapist is to provide a brave space that is non-judgmental. Many clients may never have had this space, and their LGBTQI identity disclosure to the therapist may be the first time this identity has ever been revealed to another human being. An AT therapist works to help the client develop acceptance and a healthy self-identity. It is essential that therapists have cultural humility and knowledge about the LGBTQI community which, allows for treatment to focus on empowerment and validation rather than shame and re-traumatization (Goodrich & Ginicola, 2017).

The *LGBTQI Workbook for CBT* includes handouts and worksheets to address a multitude of self-growth goals. Tips, tools, activities, and practical cognitive and behavioral exercises and homework will be included within this workbook's handouts and worksheets. The handouts and worksheets are designed to give the reader or clinician a practical tool kit for self-assessment, cognitive exercises, behavioral activities, psychoeducational tools, and therapist resources. The tools from this workbook can be used for self-reflection, in session with a therapist, in a group setting, as homework assignments, or adapted as part of intake materials. The handouts and worksheets in this workbook were designed with the rationalization of inclusion for sexual minorities in mainstream therapeutic literature. The short exercises and activities within the worksheets and handouts were designed with the intention to increase positive motivation and self-awareness, thus helping us to experience a new way of thinking, feeling, and behaving.

The workbook is divided into five parts with an icon to accompany to help the reader quickly identify the type of handout or worksheet. There is no one correct way to utilize this workbook. Clinicians can incorporate a combination of handouts and worksheets into a client's treatment plan and intervention. The reader or therapist and client can select the handouts and worksheet that work best with the identified individualized treatment plan or goal target. There is no one direction needed for this workbook; use the handouts and worksheets in the order and combination one sees as the best fit.

The first part is **Self-assessment Handouts and Worksheets**, which includes activities and exercises designed to help the reader and clinician explore the issues needing attention. The activities are designed to assess motivation, readiness for change, increase insights into current functioning, and goal setting. Change is difficult, and these practical exercises are designed to bring focus on positive change thinking and positive change behaviors – increasing the adaptive functioning and decreasing the maladaptive.

The second part of this workbook is **Cognitive Handouts and Worksheets**, which includes multiple activities and exercises designed to help the reader discover their patterns of thinking. The goal is to connect how these patterns of thinking, both positive and negative, influence one's feelings and emotions and subsequently, one's behavior. The handouts and worksheets will help identify positive versus negative thinking patterns; they will help identify common mistakes we make in our rational thinking. The ABC technique will help the reader identify thoughts, evaluate the truth and accuracy to the belief of those thoughts, and develop more positive emotional consequences. Cognitive techniques are designed to facilitate feeling better emotionally by changing the way one thinks (cognition) about an experience.

The third part of this workbook is **Behavioral Handouts and Worksheets**, which includes the exercises and activities designed to facilitate the learning of how to increase positive behaviors. Tools included in this part of the workbook are mindfulness practices, behavioral enhancement techniques, relaxation training skills, and grounding techniques.

The fourth part of this workbook is **Psychoeducational Handouts and Worksheets**, which includes information designed to facilitate the knowledge of how to change faulty thinking and increase positive behaviors. Tools included in this part of the workbook focus on education on LGBTQI history, handouts that address how to find an affirming therapist, and infographics for LGBTQI identity and nutrition are provided. Health affirming checklists are in the Part 4 toolbox as well.

The fifth part of this workbook is **Therapist Handouts and Worksheets**, which includes information, tools, worksheets, handouts, and forms to assist the therapist in the delivery of effective and sensitive services. Part 5 of the toolkit includes handouts and worksheets designed primarily for the therapist. Tool includes multiple checklists to assess trauma-informed approaches to client care, therapist tips for work within the LGBTQI community, handouts on AT, common therapist errors, and conversion therapy education. AT progress notes, biological-psychological-social AT assessment, and resources can be found in the Appendix.

The creative application of CBT techniques for the LGBTQI community in this workbook is highlighted in the multiple exercises and activities intended to increase positive thinking and new adaptive behaviors. The workbook is designed to gain insight through self-reflection and through brief goal-directed activities and exercises to help reach personal goals and objectives. The key to cognitive and behavioral change is routine practice and homework to shape new behaviors. Behaviors are learned, and with homework, they can be unlearned. Rehearsal can allow for positive behaviors to replace maladaptive old patterns. Personal rewards are important to receive to continue to keep the motivation for growth progression. This workbook's intent is to promote self-awareness, reduce maladaptive coping, increase positive thinking, and increase positive emotional outcomes in life.

TERMING CBT

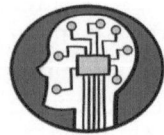

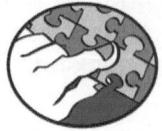

CBT 101:

- Helps you develop new coping skills.
- Improves communication in relationships.
- Challenges and conquers fears.
- Assists in developing mindfulness skills.
- Enriches self-esteem and enhances self-efficacy.
- Confronts irrational and maladaptive thought patterns.
- Creates a life worth living.
- CBT is a collaborative therapy where clients explore thoughts, emotions, and behaviors.
- CBT's central concept is you feel the way you think.
- Assists with goal setting (behavioral) and problem-solving (cognitive) skills (Beck, 2020).
- Refer to the Mental Mistakes (Cognitive Distortions) handout in Part 2 for more information on the most common patterns of negative thinking that trap us and get us stuck in maladaptive patterns which in turn can have significant impact upon emotions and behaviors.
- Refer to the ABC Technique and East vs. West Thinking handouts in Part 2 for your lists of positive beliefs, cognitions, and thoughts. Use these positive beliefs, cognitions, and thoughts, to replace old and faulty beliefs, cognitions, and thoughts that are maladaptive.

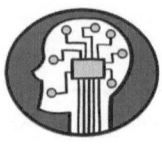

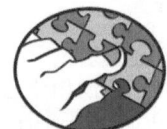

CBT Science:

- CBT is eclectic and incorporates a range of therapies and clinical techniques.
- Ongoing research continues to demonstrate that CBT is effective for a range of mental health issues.
- The therapeutic approach has been studied more than any other intervention.
- The popularity of CBT is resulting in more discovery about which aspects of the treatment are most useful for different types of human beings like LGBTQI people, people of color, genderqueer/non-binary/gender nonconforming (GNC) individuals, military service members, couples, people living with disabilities, families, members of the Neurodiversity Movement, caretakers, and others that are marginalized and may lack a voice in the dominate mainstream narrative of CBT research.
- People living with anxiety and depression stay well longer with CBT therapy.
- The strong psychoeducational component in this intervention is believed to be the positive result in CBT.
- CBT encourages the client to become their own therapist, which encourages being goal-focused, become generally short-term oriented, and take solution-focused behavioral action steps.

- CBT as a standalone intervention can be beneficial. Medication intervention (if needed), along with CBT has been shown to produce optimal mental health outcomes for those it was studied upon (Beck, 2020).

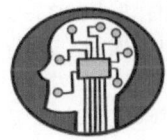

CBT Terms:

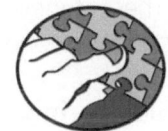

- **Cognitive (C):** A mental process like thinking that includes all the components of the mind, such as dreams, memories, attention, and thoughts.
- **Behavior (B):** Is the activity or output that one does. This includes overt behavior, as well as inaction or avoidance.
- **Therapy (T):** Describes a form of treatment that is systematically aimed at mental health symptom relief or to combat an issue through solution focused approaches.
- **Activating Event (A):** "A" is often the "trigger." The ABC format helps to break down issues and to gain an understanding of emotional challenges. The activating event can be a real external event or internal event in ones' mind, such as a memory or dream.
- **Belief (B):** Beliefs are the meanings one attaches to external and internal events or triggers. Beliefs include thoughts, rules for life, and expectations from one's culture and geography.
- **Consequences (C):** Emotions are consequences. Behaviors and physical sensations can accompany different emotions.
- **Automatic Thoughts:** A thought, image, or memory that instantly "jumps" into your mind and causes a specific emotion to be experienced and a behavior may occur in response.
- **Cognitive Distortion:** A feature of the mind which convinces us of something that isn't really true. They are inaccurate thoughts that are reinforced by negative thinking and negative emotions. See Cognitive Distortions Checklist handout.
- **Mental Mistakes (Thinking Errors):** Missteps in thinking patterns that we all make sometimes. We often jump to conclusions or assume the worst has happened when thinking errors occur. Similar to Cognitive Distortions.
- **Rules and Assumptions:** Are learned and social-culturally constructed. CBT aims to help one become more aware of their own rules and assumptions and how these contribute to a pattern of negative automatic thoughts in emotionally triggering situations.
- **Core Beliefs:** Core beliefs usually develop early in life and are the deepest cognitions that reflect rigid and absolute notions about yourself, others, and the environment. They may be more challenging to shift versus *rules* or *assumptions*.
- **Thought Recording:** With homework and rehearsal, one can become skilled at using the thought recording technique to document, question, and evaluate one's automatic thoughts and reduce emotional distress.
- **Behavioral Experiments (BE):** Powerful CBT tool for questioning and evaluating underlying assumptions and core beliefs that tests their validity. BE requires that one "test out" new ways of thinking by doing something differently. BE asks one to bring about the feared situation and confirm if what one fears actually occurred. Then, should the feared outcome occur, the experiments will also enable one's ability to cope with the situation. This level of BE is only recommended

when stable coping skills are in place, and a network of social supports is readily accessible. Please conduct experiments that you think you are ready for and be aware of what is your real historical and/or personal trauma. It is essential you have developed strategies to cope. There is a wide range of possible outcomes from these types of experiments and doing psychotherapy with a licensed professional in one's region may help strengthen one's coping skills along with homework.

- **Self-Monitoring:** Involves routinely monitoring one's moods or feelings on a daily basis, rating them on a scale from 0 to 5 or 0 to 100; monitoring symptoms of the issue in specific situations; and scheduling activities or monitoring one's progress with a behavioral goal.
- **Scheduling Activities:** CBT asks for one to schedule both pleasurable activities and life skills tasks for the upcoming day, week, month, year, or five years. Automatic thoughts are recorded during daily or weekly activities to help identify cognitive distortions.
- **Socratic Questioning:** Term was named after Socrates (c. 470–399 BCN) who encouraged a method of thought and questioning that enables us to examine ideas logically, and to determine the validity of these ideas. Using this method, CBT clinicians guide their clients to explore complex ideas, to uncover the truth of things, to reveal the nature of issues and problems, and to explore the rationale behind assumptions and rules using this tool.
- **Hot Thoughts (Cognitions):** The automatic thoughts most connected to moods. They are the thoughts that elicit an intense emotional charge such as anger or euphoria.
- **Mood Check:** This can include the use of scales to assess depression, anxiety, or other clinical issues. The client and therapist use the mood check tool in session and in-between sessions to check to see if mood improves from session to session.
- **Homework:** Assigning this in-between session work can help clients practice new skills during the week. Homework and skill rehearsal are critical components of CBT (Beck, 2020).

CBT Resource Box

- Academy of Cognitive Therapies
- Association for Behaviour and Cognitive Therapies
- Albert Ellis Institute
- British Association for Behavioural and Cognitive Psychotherapies
- National Alliance on Mental Illness (NAMI)
- National Institute of Mental Health (NIMH)
- Substance Abuse and Mental Health Services Administration (SAMHSA)
- WebMD
- Psychology Today
- International Centre for Excellent in Emotionally Focused Therapy (ICEEFT)
- Centers for Disease Control (CDC)
- Eye Movement Desensitization and Reprocessing International Association (EMDRIA)
- American Psychological Association (APA)
- The Beck Institute for CBT

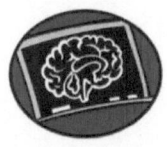 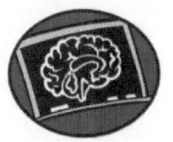

Terming LGBTQI

Always be mindful that language and terminology are ever evolving. There are infinite possibilities regarding the evolution of LGBTQI terminology, bearing it remains inclusive and affirming in nature and tone. This handout contains several websites that provided psychoeducation resources on LGBTQI terminology and regularly updated their information.

LGBTQI Resource Box

- LGBTQIA+ Glossary of Terms for Health Care Teams published by the National LGBTQIA+ Health Education Center
- LGBTQ+ Glossary published by It Gets Better
- LGBTQIA Resource Center Glossary published by LGBTQIA Resource Center
- Glossary of LGBTQ+ Vocabulary Definitions published by Its Pronounced Metrosexual

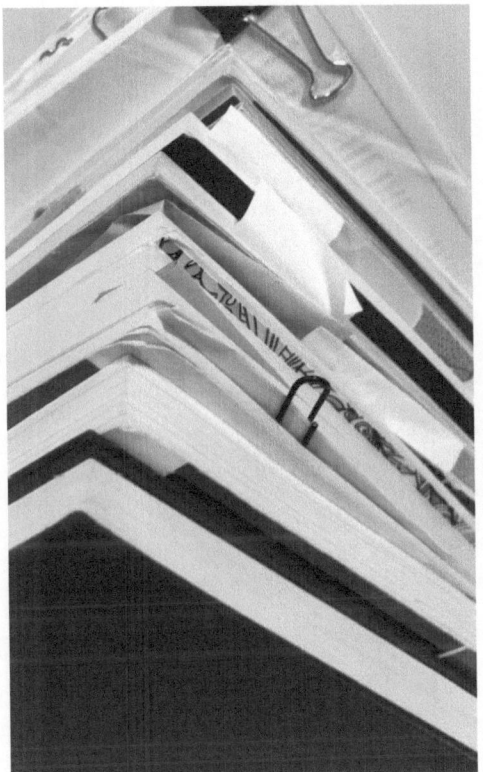

List 3 terms you were unfamiliar with:

List 3 terms that you could conversate comfortably using:

List 3 terms that would make you feel uncomfortable to use:

Part 1

Self-Assessment Handouts and Worksheets

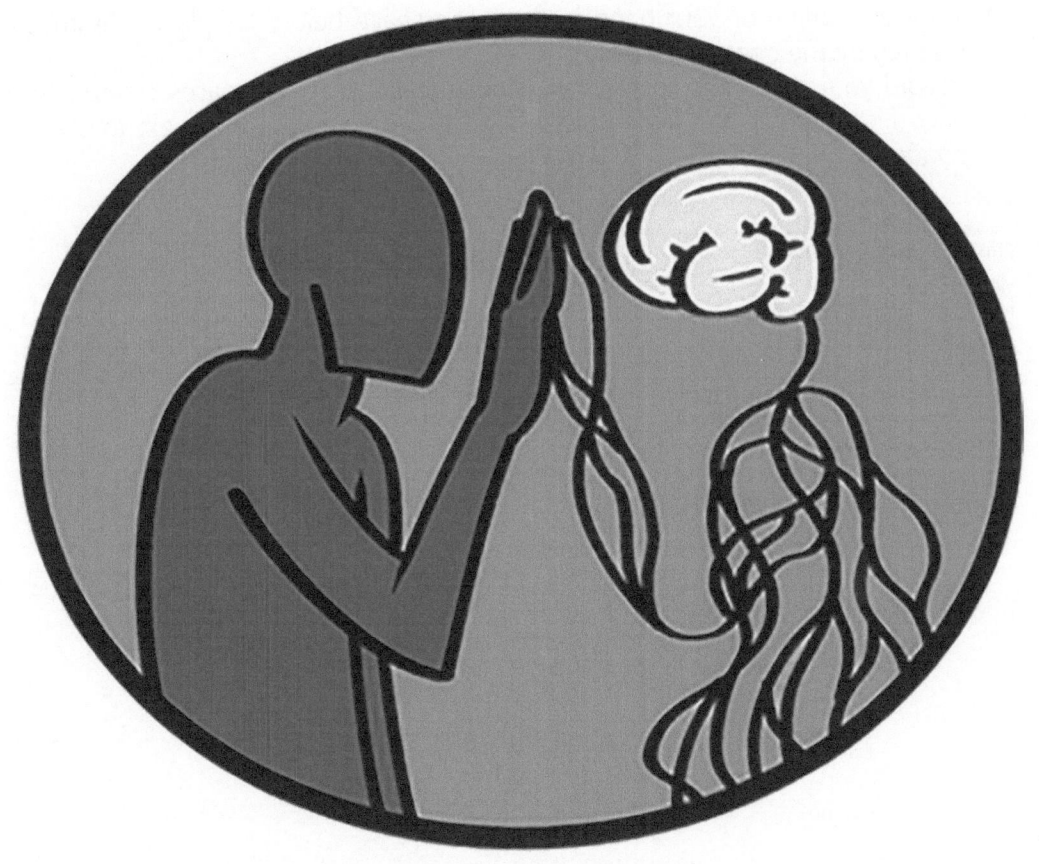

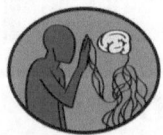 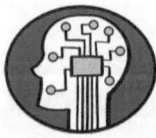 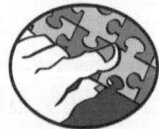

FIRSTHAND SELF-ASSESSMENT

Directions:

- Trace an outline of your hand in the open space below (or place five images inspired by the questions below);
- Record your responses to the following questions in the spaces created from each finger within the traced outline (or record your response next to the five images).

Pinkie Finger	Ring Finger	Middle Finger	Pointer Finger	Thumb
What are you here to change?	Who do you love? What do you want from relationships?	Who do you admire? Your role models?	What brings you joy? Your favorite activity?	Who are you? Who do you wish to become?

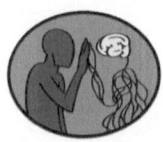 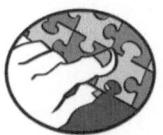

ISLANDS AND STONES GOAL SETTING

Directions: Select three goals you wish to address, and write them down on the "islands" below. These "islands" in this metaphor are what you are working or hopping towards. For each goal, break down how you will achieve this goal into three objectives. Objectives are smaller bite-sized steps that will get you to your goal or the island. Objectives are the "hopping stones" you will take to get to your "island."

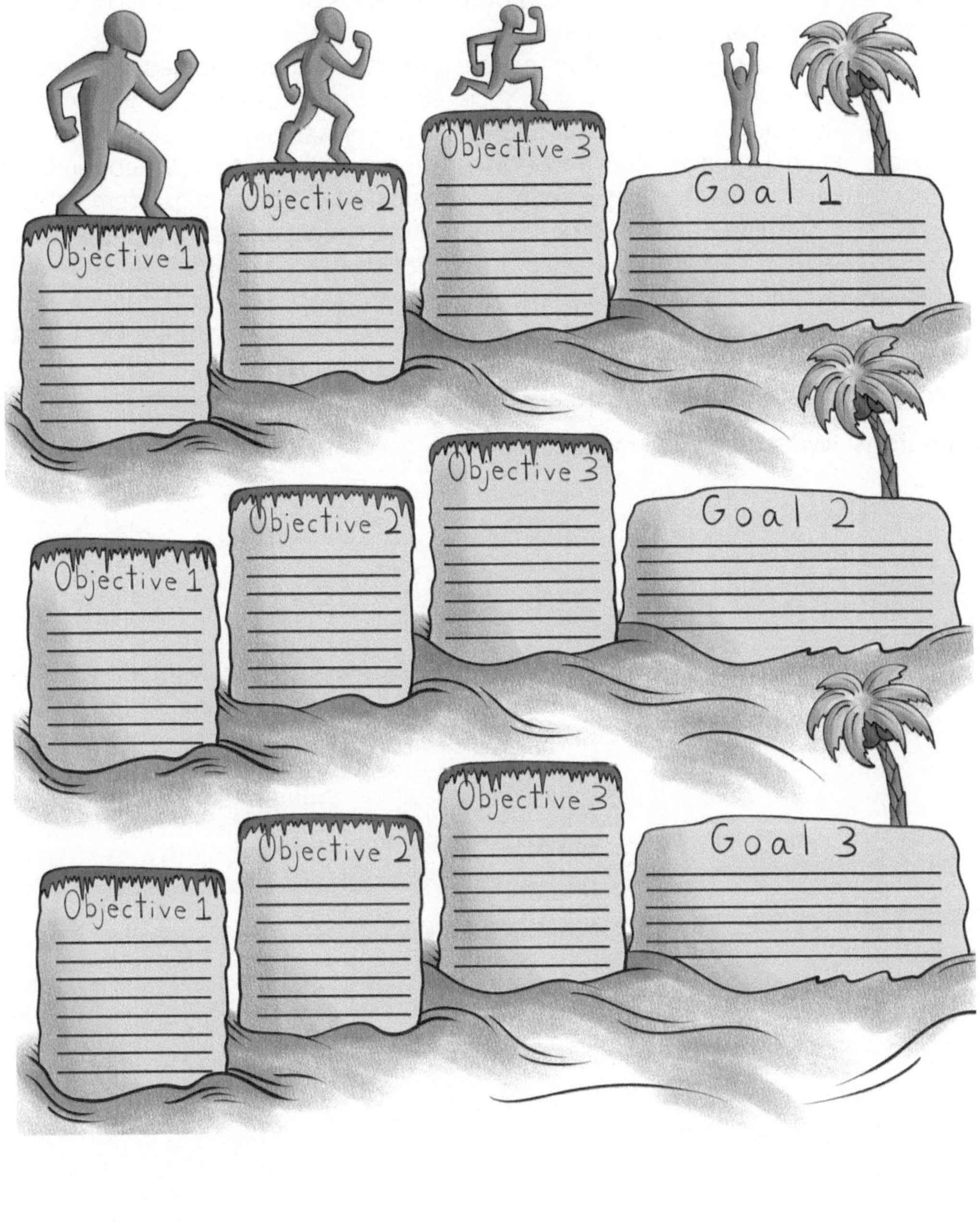

Objective 1

Objective 2

Objective 3

Goal 1

Objective 1

Objective 2

Objective 3

Goal 2

Objective 1

Objective 2

Objective 3

Goal 3

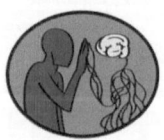

INTERSECTIONALITY GEM

Intersectionality is a framework and tool for assessment (Crenshaw, 1989). It supports conceptualizing a person, community, or social problem as distressed by a multitude of discrimination and oppression. It simultaneously considers human beings as being dynamic gemstones with multiple facets of identity. It is these facets or overlapping identities and experiences that must be assessed for in order to understand the complexity of prejudices individuals and communities face every day. For the LGBTQI community, intersectionality provides a framework to address sexual identity, gender, sex, and assigned sex at birth, but incorporates all facets of identity when considering the entire person in any given context.

Intersectional theory asserts that people are often disadvantaged by multiple sources of oppression: skin color (race), socio-economic status (SES), gender identity, sexual identity (orientation), religion and spirituality, sex, assigned sex at birth, first language, national origin, culture and ethnicity, ability, and age, to just mention a few identity markers. Intersectionality recognizes that identity markers (e.g., "female" and "black" and "lesbian" and "mother") do not exist independently of each other. Please go back and view the Audrey Lorde illustration; she held all these identities to be her own simultaneously and dynamically. Crenshaw (1989) in the seminal work defining the theory, postulates that each identity marker informs the others, often creating a complex convergence of oppression and marginalization.

Who are you? What kind of gem are you? Ruby, Sapphire, or Emerald?

Directions: Write out your identities on the gem outline and answer the four questions:

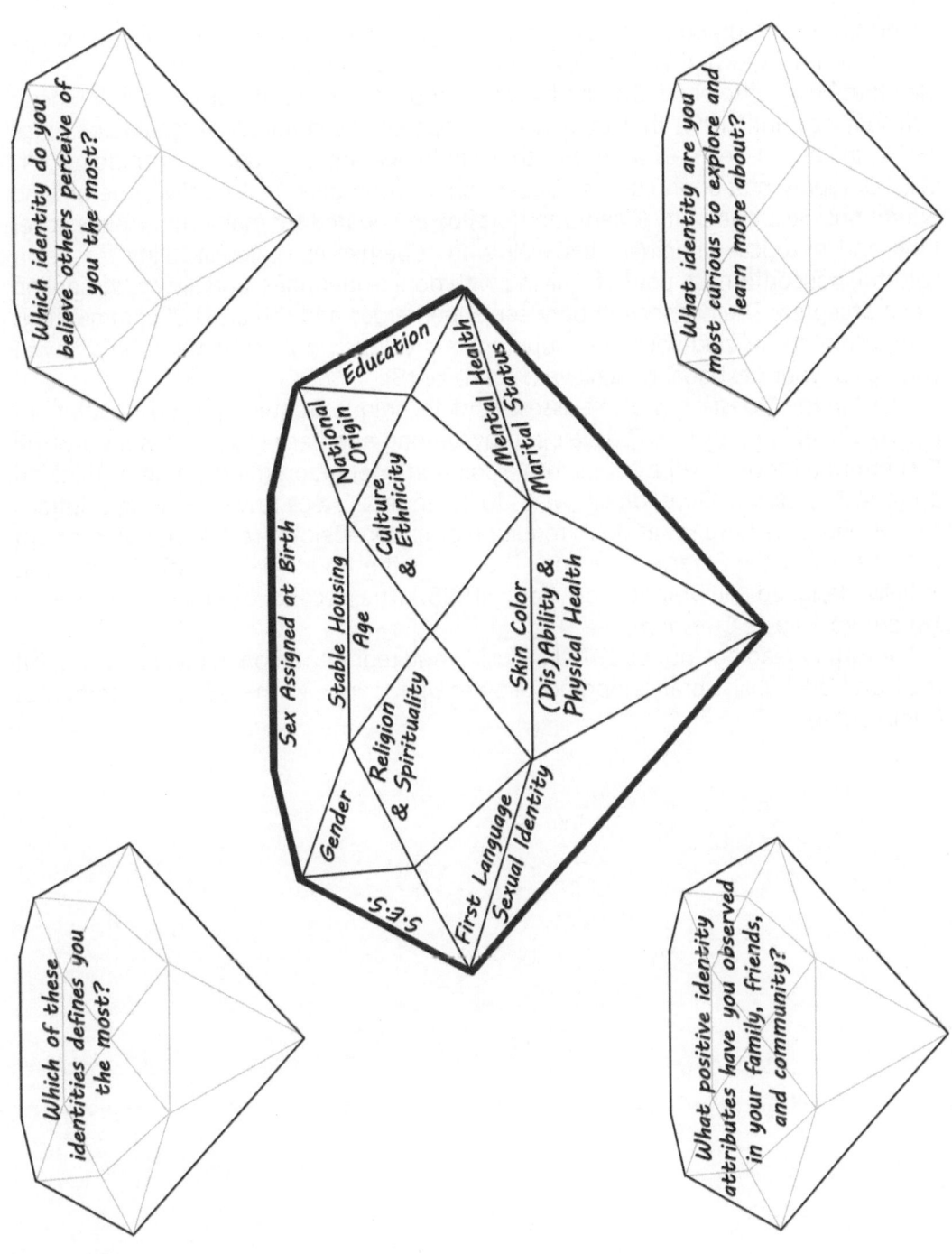

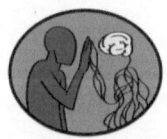

SUPERHERO MIRACLE QUESTION

Comic books and graphic novels have always given the LGBTQI community icons and heroic stories to escape within. For many in the community, superheroes model the idea that being different is OK; the fantasy world created allows for these differences.

It was not until 1992 that there was an openly gay comic book character. Since 1954, there had been an authority that controlled strict guidelines forbidding any LGBTQI representation in comics. Queer comics have been historically underground operations. Sexual identity (orientation) has been debated for many superheroes over time and historical campiness fits well with superheroes generalizability for being colorful, nonconformist, powerful, living with double identities, and always struggling to be accepted. The connection between superheroes and the LGBTQI community is compelling. Visualizing your own superpowers will be an inspiration to help power you up for your next goal to achieve (Pagan, 2018).

The *Miracle Question* is a self-assessment technique frequently used in Solution-Focused Brief Therapy (SFBT) developed by DeJong and Berg (1998). It is a powerful CBT-informed tool. It helps get us into a solution orientation mind-frame or thinking pattern. The *Miracle Question* allows us to begin small steps toward finding solutions to challenges we have set as goals requiring attention. Below are two self-assessment exercises using the *Miracle Question*. The first is the traditional *Miracle Question* as initially designed by DeJong and Berg (1998). The second example is a *LGBTQI Superhero Miracle Question*.

For further reading about LGBTQI inclusion and representation in comic books, visit the New York Public Library's blog post Power Up for Pride With LGBTQ+ Superheroes (June, 2018).

The Traditional *Miracle Question* (DeJong & Berg, 1998):

Now, I want to ask you a strange question. Suppose that while you were sleeping tonight and the entire house is quiet, a miracle happens. The miracle is that the problem which brought you here is solved. However, because you're sleeping, you don't know that the miracle has happened. So, when you wake up tomorrow morning, what will be different that will tell you a miracle has happened and the problem which bought you here is solved?

(pp. 77–78)

Directions: Consider the question above and reflect, with text or images, etc., on the following questions in the spaces on the puzzle pieces below:

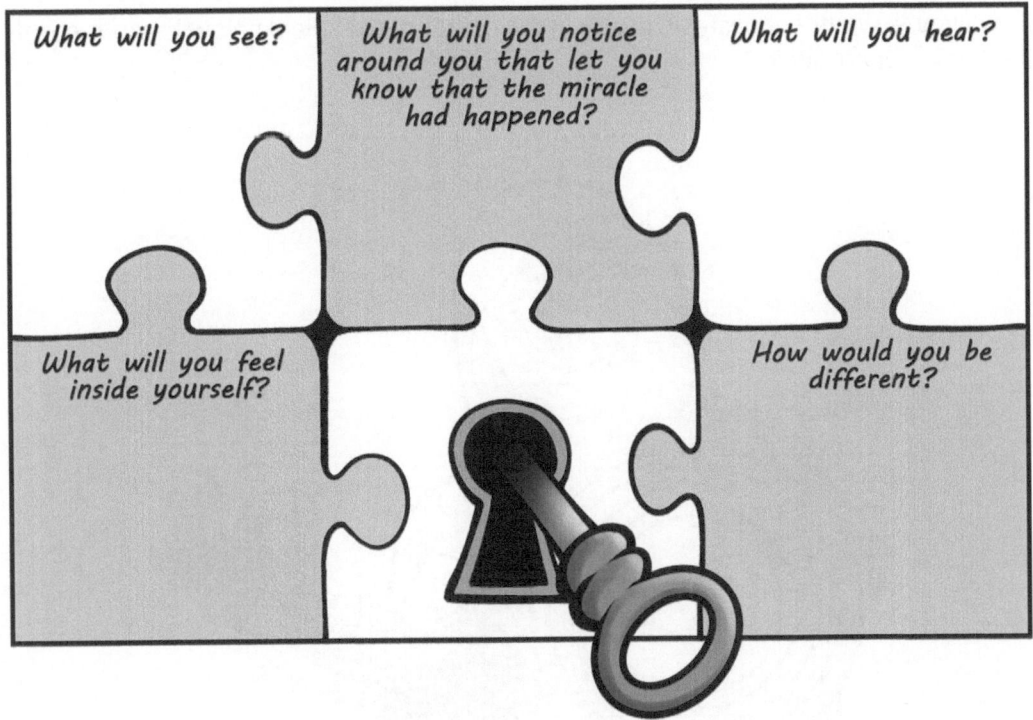

The *LGBTQI Superhero Miracle Question* (An Adaptation of the Original):

Suppose you could drink from the fountain that gives you one superhero strength or ability to do something supernatural. Drinking from the fountain one evening would give you a supernatural power or superhero ability the next morning after you awoke. The new superpower would provide you with strength and fill you with courage. This strength in-turn would then allow you to take precise steps towards overcoming your challenge.

- What kind of almost supernatural power would you need to overcome your challenge?
- When you awake with your new superpower envision your challenge being resolved – what would be different if this occurred?
- How would you handle the new situation? How might you imagine coping?
- Please talk about the details of your entire story, including compelling step-by-step details.
- Draw a symbol or paste an image in the center of the shield below that represents your superpower.

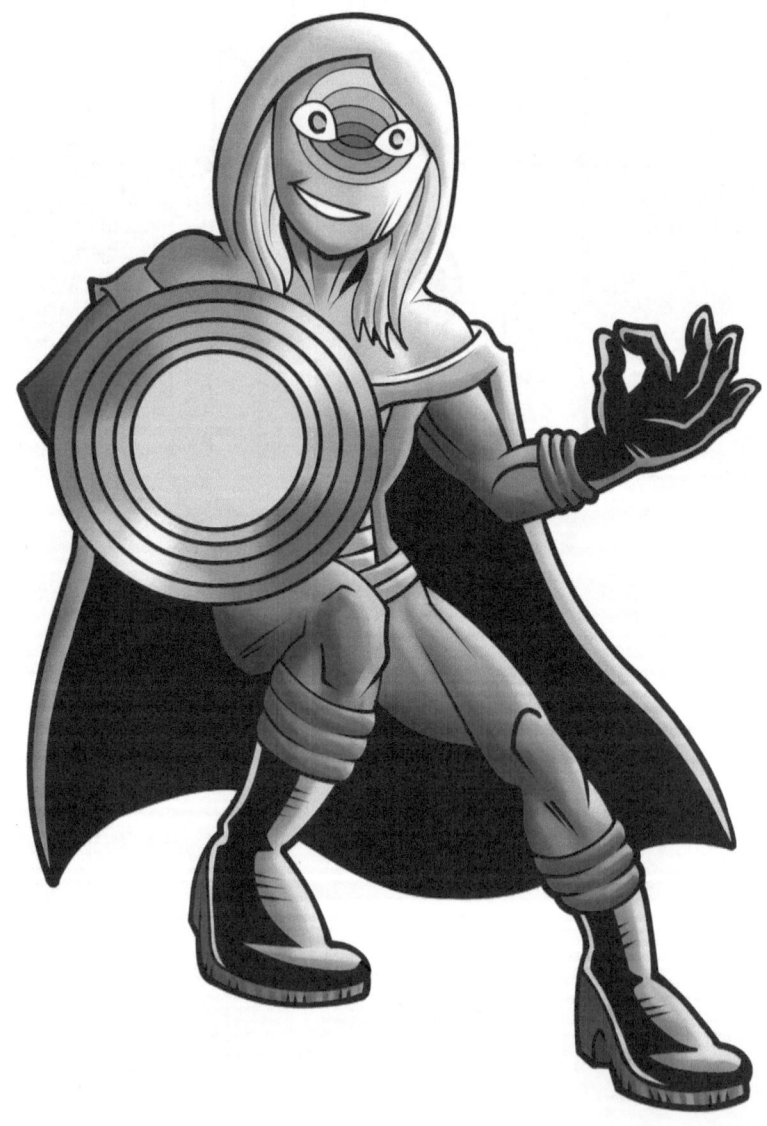

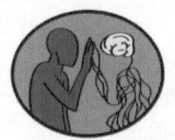 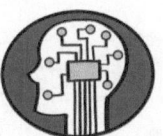

EMOTIONAL COLOR CORAL

This worksheet is like a bright underwater thermostat for your emotional self-reflection while grounding yourself emotionally with active coloring behavior. The Atlas of Emotions website is a cognitive and self-reflective tool supported by the Dalai Lama that can assist you in identifying emotional states of mind. The LGBTQI rainbow pride flag colors are often associated with the community in a positive light.

Directions: First, begin by identifying which emotions are at the root of your current state of mind. The common root emotions (dependent upon culture) listed in the coral are disgust, anger, enjoyment, fear, and sadness. Some emotions are often then experienced in response to earlier emotions. We feel anger first, then feel shame because we responded with anger. Using the Atlas of Emotions website, write down the emotions you notice in the coral. Color the section of coral with the color you identify with that emotion. Another option could be to access the core list of emotions from social work researcher and storyteller Dr. Brené Brown on her website under downloads.

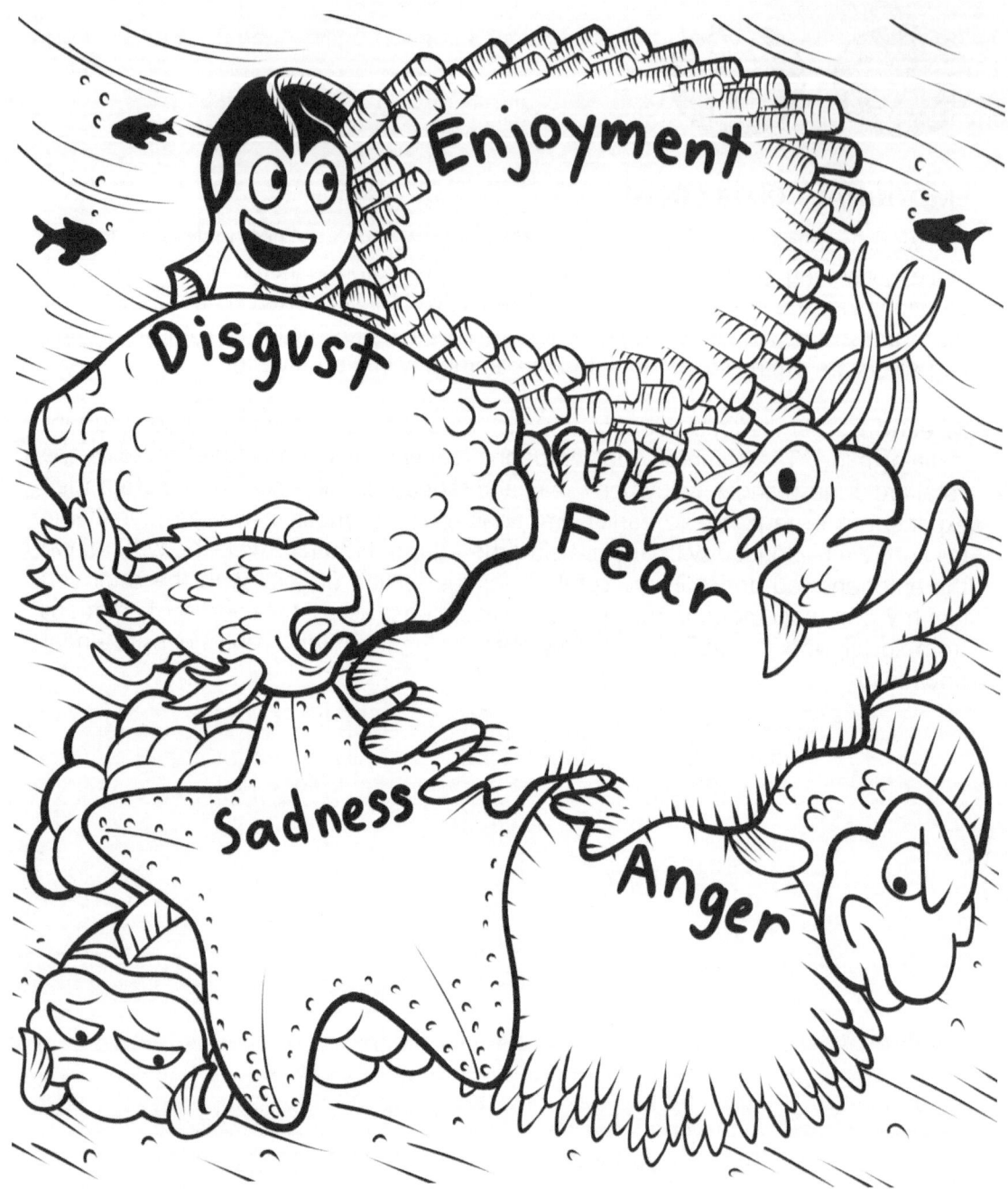

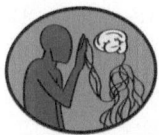 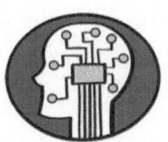 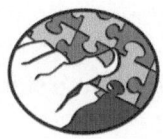

LGBTQI HIERARCHY

Maslow's (1987) famous hierarchy is a tool for assessment. For the LGBTQI community, it can help assess for the basic needs of any individual. Many, because of an LGBTQI identity, often do not have even their basic needs (e.g., affirming housing and food) met because of rejection, homophobia, transphobia, biphobia, and heterosexism. In Los Angeles, 40% of homeless youth identify as LGBTQ. LGBTQ young adults are more than twice as likely to experience homelessness compared to non-LGBTQ young adults in the USA (Tambe & Rice, 2018). There are health-related problems when one can't access a gender-neutral bathroom. Refuge Restrooms is a web application resource helping to address this health-related issue. Refuge Restroom seeks to provide safe restroom access for trans, intersex, and genderqueer/non-binary/GNC individuals.

Below is Maslow's (1987) pyramid with the revised eight stages of hierarchical development. Review the definitions for each of the stage's benchmarks in the pyramid below, and self-reflect on whether you have mastered the "proposed" tasks of the stage.

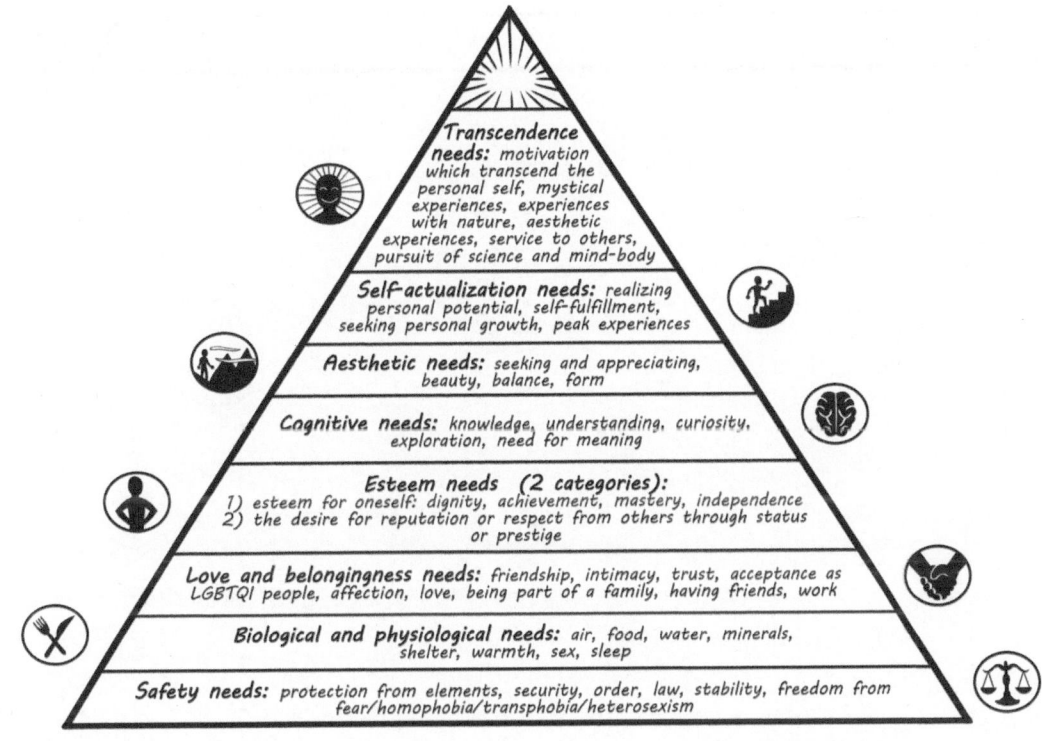

19

Directions: Fill in the blank pyramid with your thoughts and identifications from your self-reflection. Make notes in the spaces below from your own personal highlights that exemplify the definitions for each of Maslow's stages.

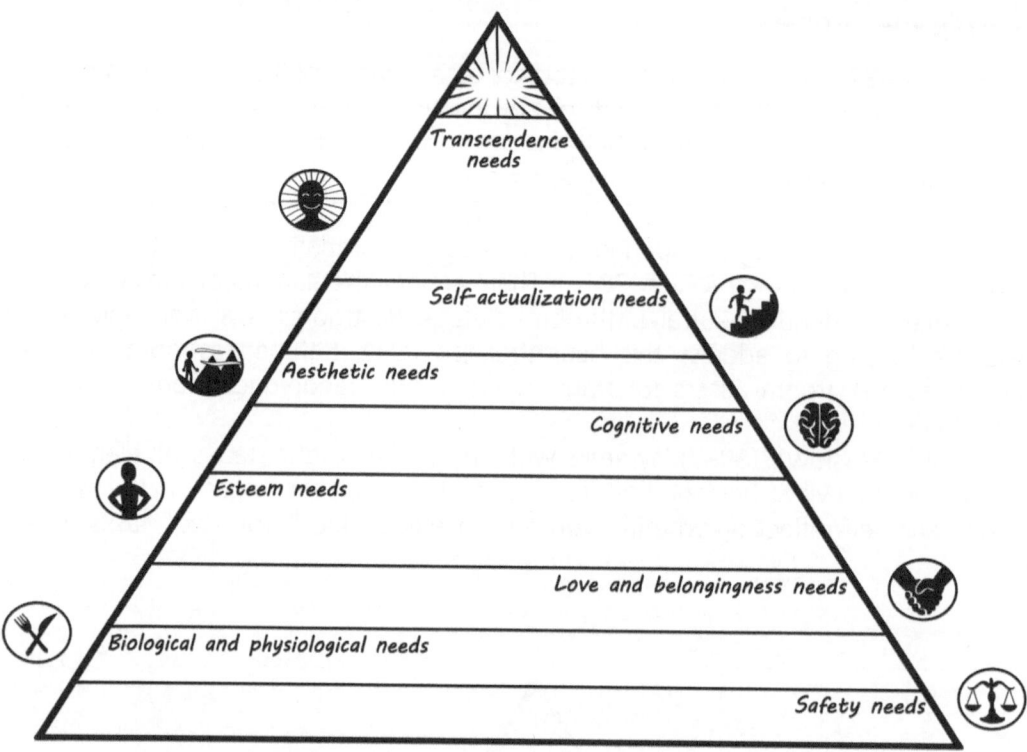

21 Characteristics of LGBTQI Self-actualizers and Those Achieving Transcendence (Maslow, 1987):

1. Self-actualizers and those members of the LGBTQI community that have achieved transcendence can tolerate uncertainty in challenging times and perceive reality efficiently (e.g., understanding the lack of legal protections for members of the LGBTQI community);
2. Accept themselves for who they are (this is tough to do regardless of your identity);
3. Spontaneous in an adaptive manner;
4. Problem-centered (e.g., not self-centered);
5. Use humor in an adaptive fashion;
6. Observe life objectively;
7. Creative and innovative;
8. Avoid radical enculturation;
9. Concerned for the welfare of humanity (e.g., why are LGBTQI teenagers at higher risk for suicide);
10. Capable of deep appreciation of basic life-experience (e.g., access to clean water);
11. Establish deep satisfying interpersonal relationships with a few people (e.g., free from intimate partner violence on the part of the victim/survivor and/or perpetrator);
12. Peak experiences (not while on substances);
13. Need for privacy (the right for any family in this country and in this world);
14. Democratic attitudes (e.g., Harvey Milk);
15. Strong moral and ethical standards;
16. Motivated by selflessness (e.g., adopting children or helping those less fortunate);
17. Mystical experiences (clarity of thought that feels as if it is from another realm);
18. Connection to nature (e.g., touring the Everglades in Florida);
19. Aesthetic experiences (e.g., hiking the Grand Canyon or Yosemite);
20. Service to the community and greater society (e.g., volunteering with Gay for Good);
21. Always acknowledging science and understanding the mind-body connection.

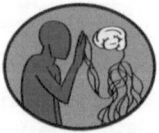 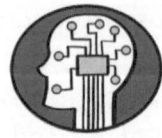 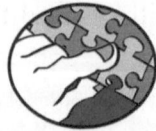

STAGES OF CHANGE LOTUS FLOWER

The lotus flower is the metaphor for change in this handout and worksheet based on the Transtheoretical Model (TTM) of change (Prochaska, Redding, & Evers, 2015). The lotus flower can be a metaphor for your life. The flower must be rooted in the mud to grow; this represents the challenges we encounter in life and as members of the LGBTQI community. The beautiful lotus flower blossoms above the water, representing the journey to overcoming our problems through finding solutions. The lotus flower opens each of its petals one by one and challenges us to become better versions of ourselves as we tackle life by setting goals and achieving objectives.

Consider these five possible steps when activating individual change. These steps may not be for everyone and may not be linear for some; they may be short or longer in timeframe. Pick one thing you wish to change. What step are you on in this goal?

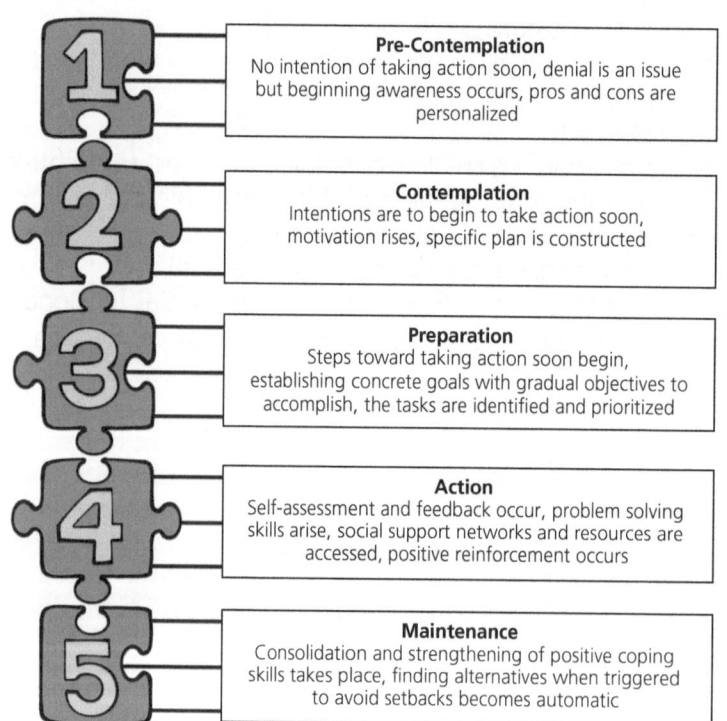

1

Pre-Contemplation
No intention of taking action soon, denial is an issue but beginning awareness occurs, pros and cons are personalized

2

Contemplation
Intentions are to begin to take action soon, motivation rises, specific plan is constructed

3

Preparation
Steps toward taking action soon begin, establishing concrete goals with gradual objectives to accomplish, the tasks are identified and prioritized

4

Action
Self-assessment and feedback occur, problem solving skills arise, social support networks and resources are accessed, positive reinforcement occurs

5

Maintenance
Consolidation and strengthening of positive coping skills takes place, finding alternatives when triggered to avoid setbacks becomes automatic

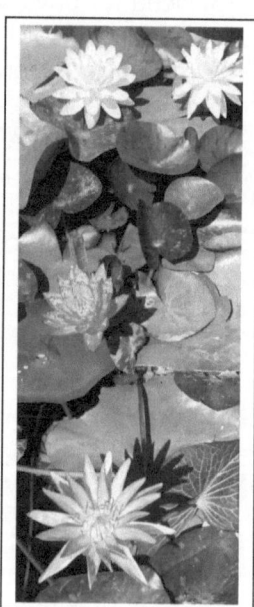

Directions: Decide which of the five steps you are currently in with your goal. The step you decide upon will be represented by the middle/center pedal below. The subsequent stages will follow on each petal in a clockwise direction. For example, if you are on step 3: action, you would place in the space of the middle/center petal below a doodle, drawing, stickers, stamps, words, or cut-and-paste printed images that represents why you are currently in this stage. Then move clockwise to complete something for each of the remaining four steps on the lotus petals.

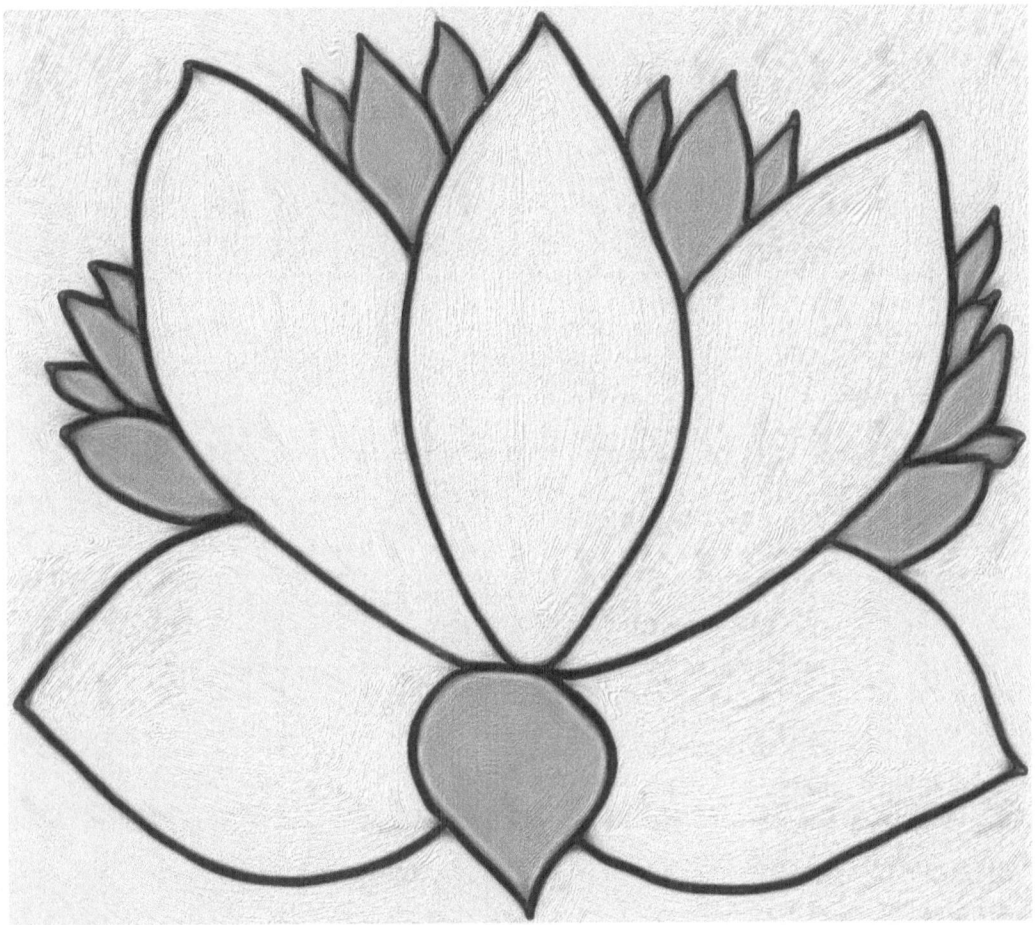

(Schott, J., 2020)

Part 2

Cognitive Handouts and Worksheets

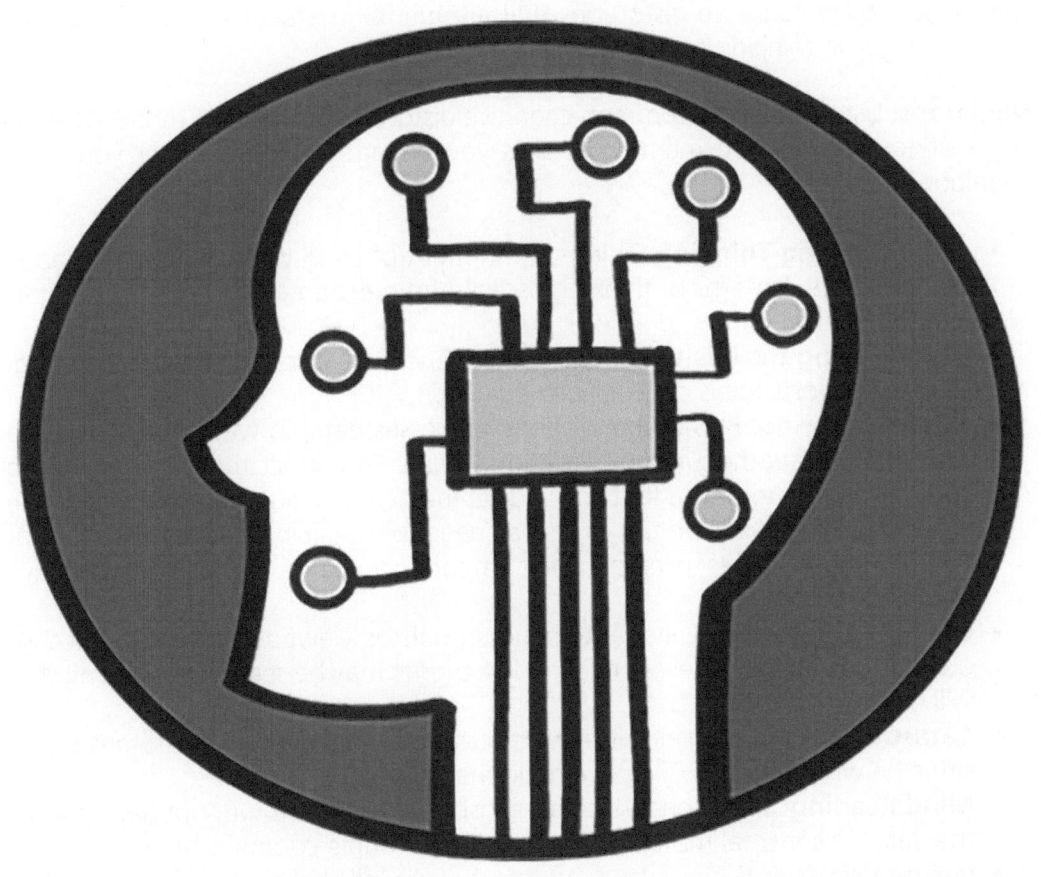

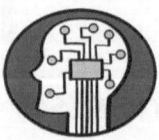

COGNITIVE DISTORTIONS CHECKLIST

Patterns of thinking are learned over time. With homework and rehearsal, we can catch and modify cognitive distortions that are mental mistakes we engage in that produce negative thinking errors.

Directions: Listed are some common cognitive distortions in the CBT model. Use the checklist to review which mental mistakes you engage in and monitor your own cognitions.

- **All-or-Nothing Thinking:** Things are thought of as all yes or all no, with no in between area. Patterns of thinking oscillate from extremes. Automatic thoughts are polarized.
- **Disqualifying the Positive:** Positive experiences are discounted and minimized. Cognitive efforts focus only on the negative.
- **Mental Filtering:** Bias in the way one processes data, in which only that data that supports the held belief is acknowledged. To correct this data-processing bias, collect the evidence that contradicts the negative automatic thoughts one is having. One pays attention to a small negative detail in an experience so that this experience takes over as great importance when having this negative automatic thought.
- **Overgeneralization:** Every automatic thought is viewed as negative because one negative trigger or event occurred. A trigger may be seen as something that will never end.
- **Catastrophizing:** Imagining the worst-case scenario. Here one assumes that a situation will be more awful or horrible than it is likely to be.
- **Mind Reading:** When one's thoughts rush to conclusions without having all of the data. This mental mistake is common with couple communication.
- **Personalization:** When events are not going well the cause is interpreted as something personal or that one is the cause of a negative event.
- **Thinking Flexibility:** When inflexible demands are placed on oneself, others, or the environment, this often means one does not adapt to reality well. Thoughts and beliefs center on "must," "should," or "need" and are challenging because they are ridged and extreme.
- **Low Frustration Tolerance or Magnifying:** Mental mistake in which one assumes that when something is difficult to tolerate, it is "devastating." Magnification of the discomfort occurs during this thinking error.
- **Emotional Reasoning:** When it is felt to be true, then it must be accepted as true unquestioned.
- **Labeling:** Cognitive process of placing negative labels on self, community, or group.
- **Blaming:** Automatically assuming the cause is oneself, and harshly takes the blame (see the Checking Toxic Shame handout for more self-assessment).

- **Fortune Telling or Crystal Ball Gazing:** Predicting future outcomes, often negative, before they have taken place. Looking into the crystal ball and making negative predictions. Maladaptive thinking occurs when one tries to guess how the future will turn out. This mental mistake keeps one from taking action (see Crystal Ball Gazing handout and worksheet).

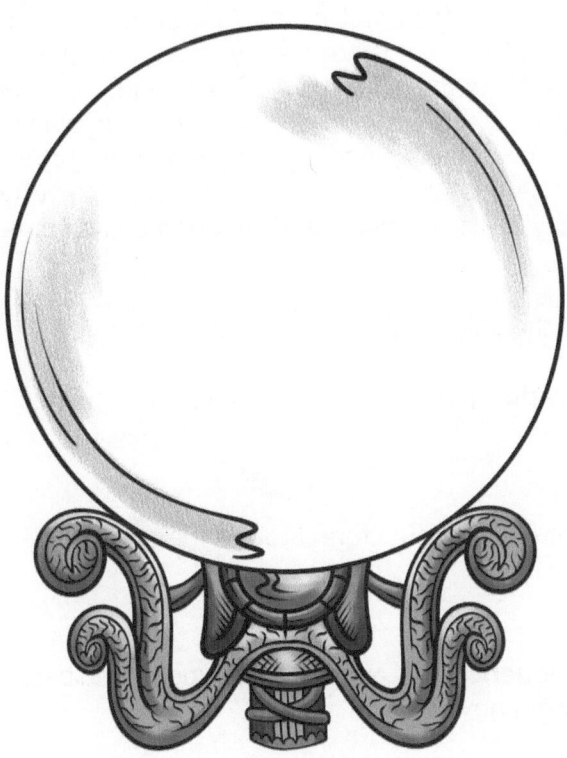

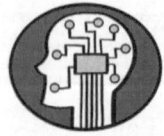 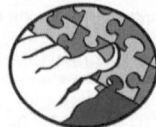

ABC TECHNIQUE

Sometimes disturbing developmental life and/or historical traumas impact members of the LGBTQI community, and it is not merely just about changing how one thinks. A critical cognitive skill is to master is the ABC Technique. The ABC Technique is one of the most popular of the CBT concepts. Often our belief (B) about what is happening around us is faulty, leading to inaccurate or unneeded emotional consequences (C). Use this worksheet to help form adaptive beliefs (B) that shed positivity or neutrality as a consequence (C) in our life each time you experience an activating (A) event.

Directions: Identify the following:

- **Stage 1: Activation (A)**, an event occurs; What happened to me?;

- **Stage 2: Belief (B)**, thoughts form around the event; What is my narrative?;

- **Stage 3: Consequences (C)**, emotions are experienced based on those thoughts; How do I feel right now?

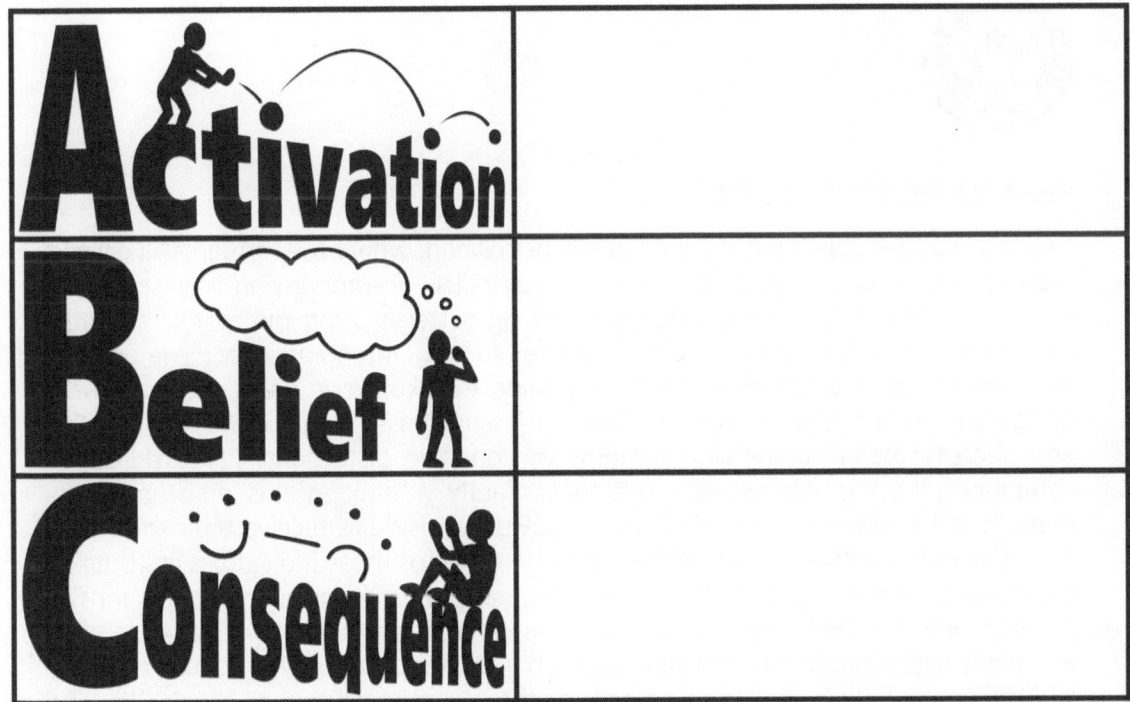

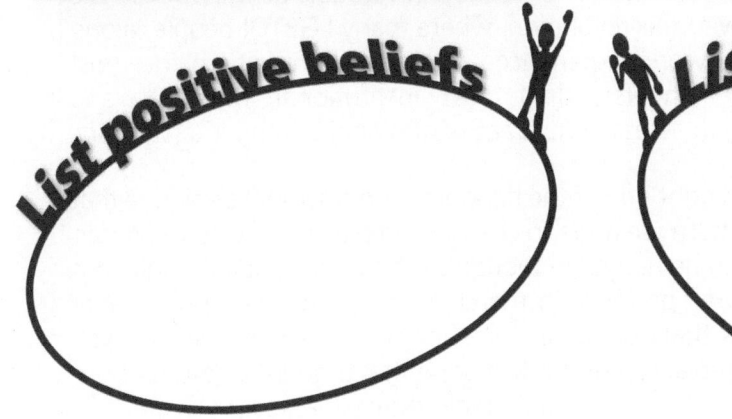

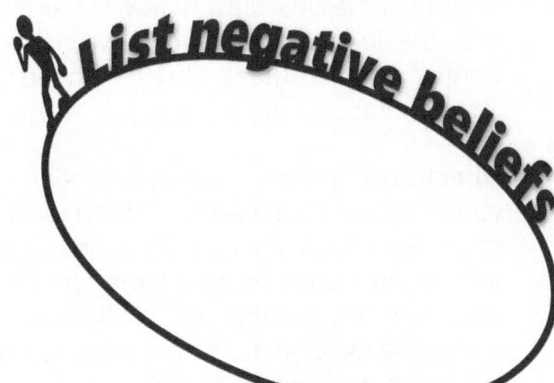

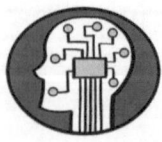

EAST VS. WEST THINKING

This tool was developed while sitting at a café in Berlin, where the former Wall divided the city in two for 28 years from 1961 to 1989. The accompanying worksheet will help to identify positive verses negative thinking patterns using the east versus west metaphor. The Berlin Wall divided so many for so long. Intending to achieve unity of mind and body, this activity is about beginning to take down walls and build new bridges in terms of thought patterns. The goal is to increase positive or neutral thinking and decrease negative thinking patterns or cognitive distortions. For the LGBTQI community, it is the heterosexist world that is faulty in thinking. It is important to be mindful of the context from which many LGBTQI individuals receive their social and cognitive programming. Much of the faulty thinking for these individuals lies outside themselves. Germany, and Berlin in particular, have been progressive systems for the advancement of LGBTQI rights in recent times. Berlin was one of the first cities to elect an openly gay mayor and historically has been a contemporary city of inclusion for the LGBTQI community. It was the epicenter of the sexual revolution of the 1920s. The atrocity of the Holocaust followed this revolution, where many LGBTQI people, along with the Jewish citizens of the world experienced a crise of humanity in the most horrific manner (Ross, 2015). Understanding one's institutional, historical, and intergenerational trauma is key in assessment, treatment planning, and intervention.

Directions: On the left side and right side of the handout, find a symbol or picture that represents this dual thinking pattern we hope to change and place it next to the photo of the Berlin Wall. It is also OK to be neutral in thoughts. This all-or-nothing thinking is a common mental mistake we all perform. In the chart, begin to write out in brief statements the negative self-talk that goes on in one's head (e.g., I am self-destructive), and at the same time, find the replacement positive or neutral thought as this thought is the true belief one should hold onto (e.g., I am practicing wellness).

Positive Cognitions:

Negative Cognitions:

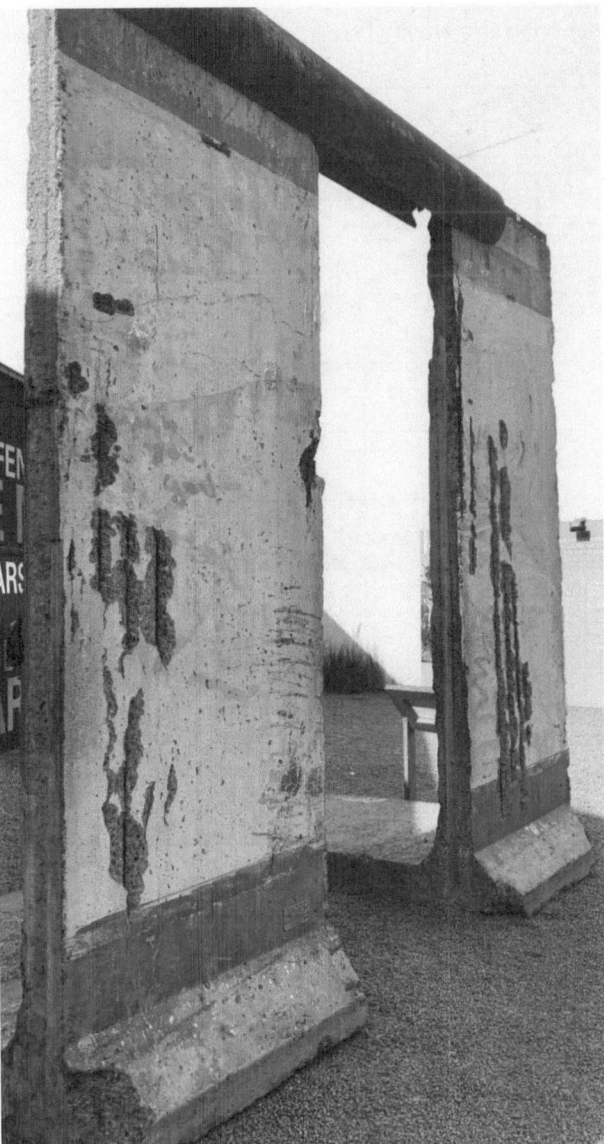

Berlin Wall at the BlackBox Cold War Museum, Berlin, Germany. July 28, 2019.

Pro-sunrise (East) with the New Thought	Con-sunset (West) with the Old Thought

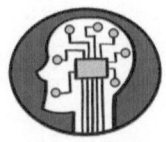 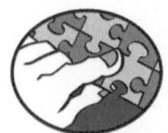

CHECKING TOXIC SHAME

An important component of a common source of shame is often related to failing in front of someone important, like your family of origin. Shame-based thinking is toxic to the mind and body. The ensuing behaviors that follow these maladaptive thought patterns are unhelpful to the LGBTQI community and human beings in general. The LGBTQI Brain handout provides us with more information on the impact of trauma. Toxic shame may be an important underlying theme in many therapy sessions, so identifying this early as a treatment goal could help you get towards resolution and increase adaptive coping skills sooner.

Consider taking the free shame test on the British Association of Anger Management website (this is only a self-assessment tool and may not be a valid measure for capturing all human being's experiences with this emotion). Check out this resource on a negative emotion typology tool hosted on the website from Delft University of Technology in the Netherlands. The tool was designed to help distinguish the nuances of our various emotions (while this handout discusses shame, it could also be used for other associated emotions like humiliation, guilt, embarrassment, and remorse).

The prior four handouts in Part 2 of this workbook directly connect to working on the goal of reducing shame, particularly the ABC Technique and East vs. West Thinking handouts and worksheets. Completing the Biological-Psychological-Social AT Assessment at the end of the workbook gives you more data for self-assessment and personal reflection, or it may provide your therapist with intake information.

The final handout in Part 2 is about channeling positive emotions and leaving the negative ones behind through the Unicorn vs. Dragon metaphor. Consider reflecting on the metaphor of the dragon when thinking about your destructive patterns of shameful thought and shame-based maladaptive behavior. The unicorn represents your positive replacement for the shame, such as pride.

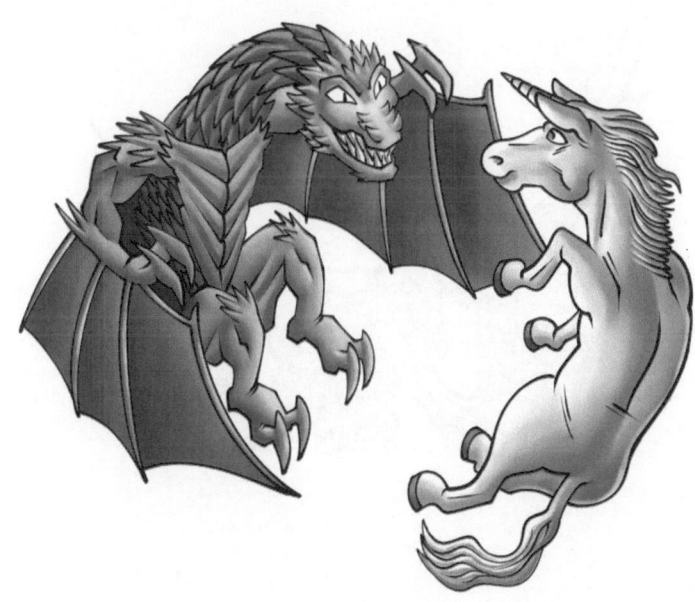

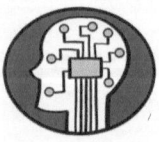

CRYSTAL BALL GAZING

Engaging in *Crystal Ball Gazing* thinking is one of the most common mental mistakes.

When we gaze into the crystal ball, we begin to think about events in the future that haven't yet occurred. We predict how the event will turn out, often with an assumption of a negative outcome. This faulty thinking leads us to give up or lose motivation because of the fear or other emotions that then lead our brain to assume these faulty predictions from the crystal ball are true, when they are not. If we are not responsible for our thinking, with this mental mistake, thoughts can also become somewhat like a self-fulfilling prophecy.

Try these strategies to break the mental mistake of fortune-telling: (1) Test out your predictions to see if they are as true as you have already assumed them to be; (2) Take a calculated risk, as it might keep life interesting; and (3) What happened to you in the past doesn't predict your future.

Directions: First, "fortune tell" with words, drawings, or images the feared future outcome in the crystal ball below.

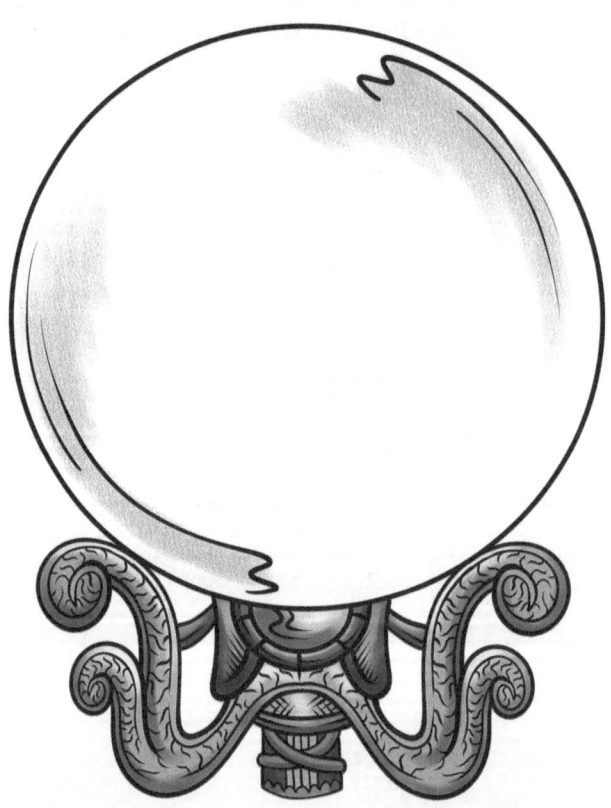

Next, write down or draw out all the events that must happen for this outcome to occur in the crystal ball below.

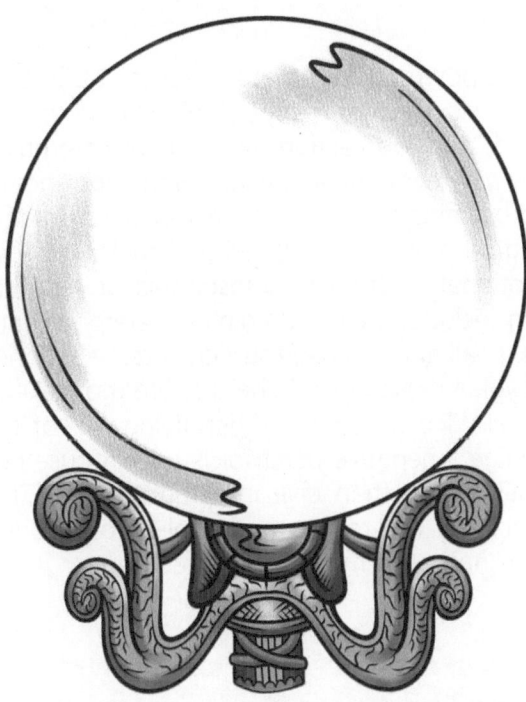

Finally, write down or draw out all the things that could occur to prevent the outcome from happening in the crystal ball below.

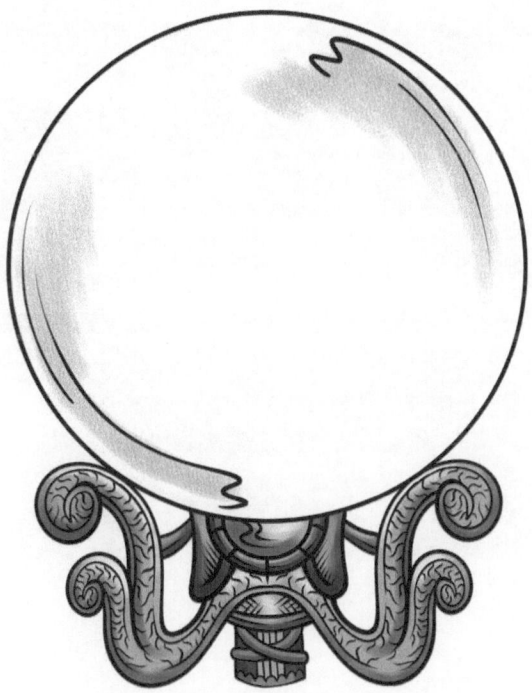

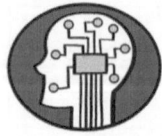 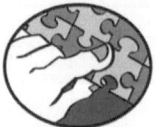

HALT TECHNIQUE

The HALT Technique is a powerful tool that has roots in the recovery community. As we learned earlier, the basic needs of many LGBTQI individuals are not met, according to the Maslow pyramid, due to rejection by family or community and homophobia and transphobia. They may cope maladaptively with substances. It is essential when accessing this tool to be mindful of the context in which many LGBTQI individuals might feel *hungry* (e.g., a teenager is bullied and their lunch is stolen daily), *angry* (e.g., a common emotional reaction to transphobia or hate crimes, murder, etc.), *lonely* (e.g., not being included in the dominant heteronormative narrative can be isolating), and *tired* (e.g., all humans need sufficient rest – see the Behavior Activation worksheet for sleep hygiene). Negative behaviors are most likely to occur when you are feeling one of the HALT conditions. By identifying one of these four conditions, when the urge to indulge a negative behavior is present, use imagery and the chart below to address HALT, rather than give into the impulse. This technique can be applied beyond the recovery community and applies to anyone seeking to improve their mental health, wellness, and mindfulness practice.

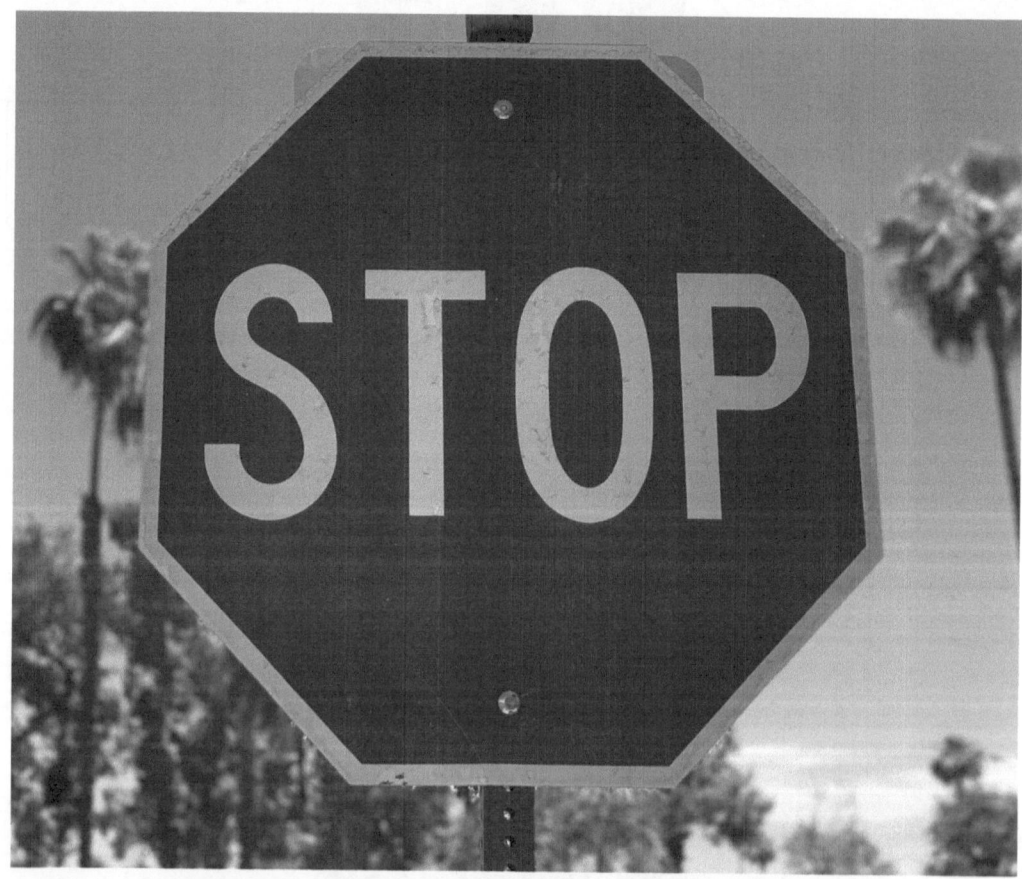

Directions: Place the photo of the stop sign in a place where you feel it will catch your attention (or any image you like that best represents this idea). This image is to remind you to check on the following four feelings: hunger, anger, lonely, and tired. In the space below, write out action steps (with or without images) you can take to positively address the four feelings when observed and experienced.

Hungry	Angry	Lonely	Tired

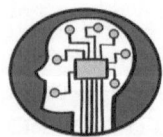 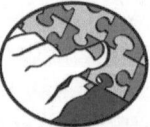

UNICORN VS. DRAGON

When anger is experienced as an emotional state, one should visualize or think of the dragon and unicorn metaphor. When our anger reacts like a dragon, we might be self-destructive and hurt others emotionally. The goal is to channel your reaction like that of the unicorn. The unicorn calmly maintains its forward direction and avoids dangerous entanglements. Fantasy creatures have always been popular in the LGBTQI community, often modeling differences are good.

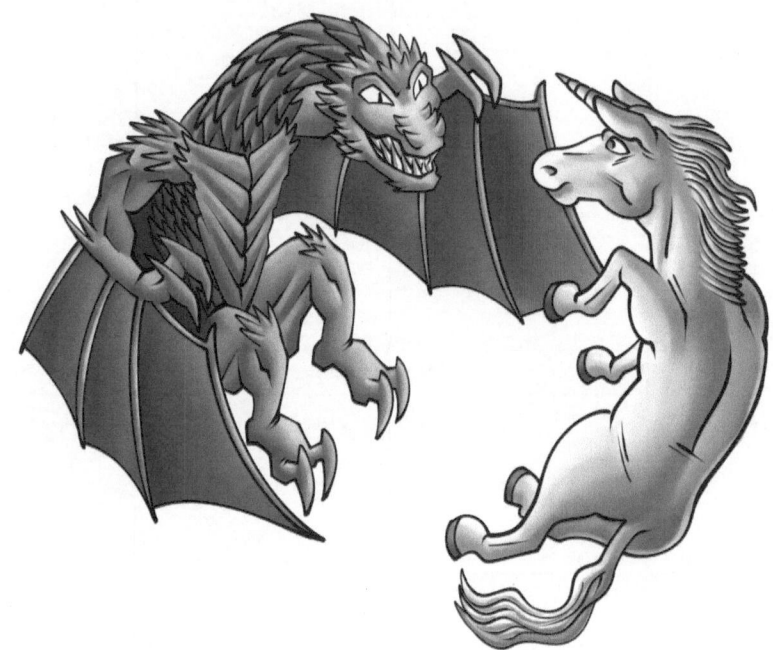

An Angry Dragon Does the Following:

1. Flaps its wings and grows bigger;
2. Breathes fire;
3. Has a scaly exterior that pushes others away;
4. Sticks out its claws;
5. Moves aggressively towards others;
6. Has piercing eyes that dilate and glare.

A Calm Unicorn Does the Following:

1. Points its horn forward and moves in a positive direction;
2. The horn gives insight and is a diamond mind or 3rd eye;
3. Gallops away from danger;
4. Remains still and silent when tense;
5. Runs with other unicorns for support;
6. Is noble and magical.

Part 3

Behavioral Handouts and Worksheets

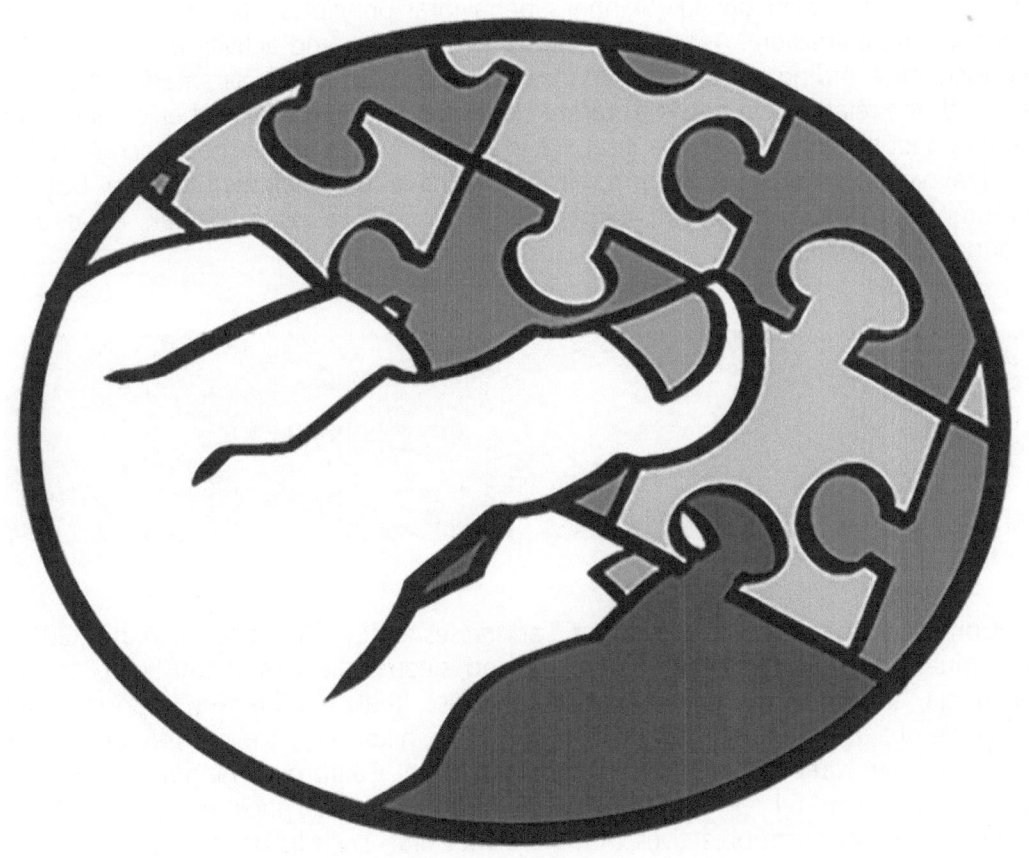

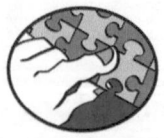

BEHAVIORAL ACTIVATION 101

Behavioral Activation (BA) is an empirically validated treatment, like CBT. The intervention is based on B.F. Skinner's behavioral principles. BA and CBT overlap substantially. Behavioral Activation includes goal setting and activity monitoring. BA consists of recording self-data via charts, handouts, worksheet, or smartphone apps to track the relationship between target behaviors, activities, and other components that impact the completion of a goal. BA is a technique to also target procrastination and avoidance. Practical elements from BA have been applied to the LGBTQI community in this workbook to target specific behavioral issues (Sudak, Majeed, & Youngman, 2014).

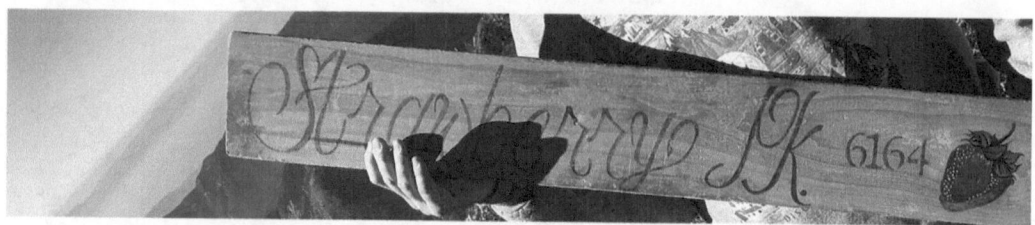

Common to most communities, Part 3 addresses topics of importance in the LGBTQI community, such as substance misuse, smoking, sleep hygiene, and nutrition (Conron, Mimiaga, & Landers, 2010). Establishing exercise goals can be very important. An example of a goal depending on ability could be to hike to the top of Strawberry Peak in the Angeles National Forest in Los Angeles County, California. The goal was to hike to the peak at 6,164 feet (Machu Pichu is 7,972 feet), but prior to this goal, there were smaller, bite-size objectives that were met first, such as hour-long walks each week, combined with at least several strenuous hikes that went up in elevation. The Goal Setting worksheet coordinates well with therapeutic work using many of the behavioral activation worksheets and grounding techniques found in Part 3 of this workbook.

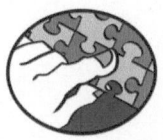

BEHAVIORAL ACTIVATION: MOTIVATING FOR AFFIRMING THERAPY

The development of a positive behavioral activation plan can help achieve a targeted goal, hopefully leading to improved mood and increased physical wellness. The goal to increase motivation to begin affirmative therapy can be broken down into smaller bite-sized objectives. List three to five options one could take to increase motivating behaviors to begin affirmative therapy. The worksheet coordinates with the LGBTQTI Affirmative Therapy handout in Part 5 of the workbook.

Goal: Increase motivating behaviors to begin affirmative therapy

Behavioral Activation Plan: List three to five behaviors related to increasing the chances of beginning this goal

---

Resource Box

- Mental Health Services at The Los Angeles LGBT Center
- Web provider directory at LGBTQ Affirmative Psychotherapy Guild of Utah
- Web provider directory at the National Queer and Trans Therapists of Color Network
- Find a therapist search feature on Psychology Today's website

---

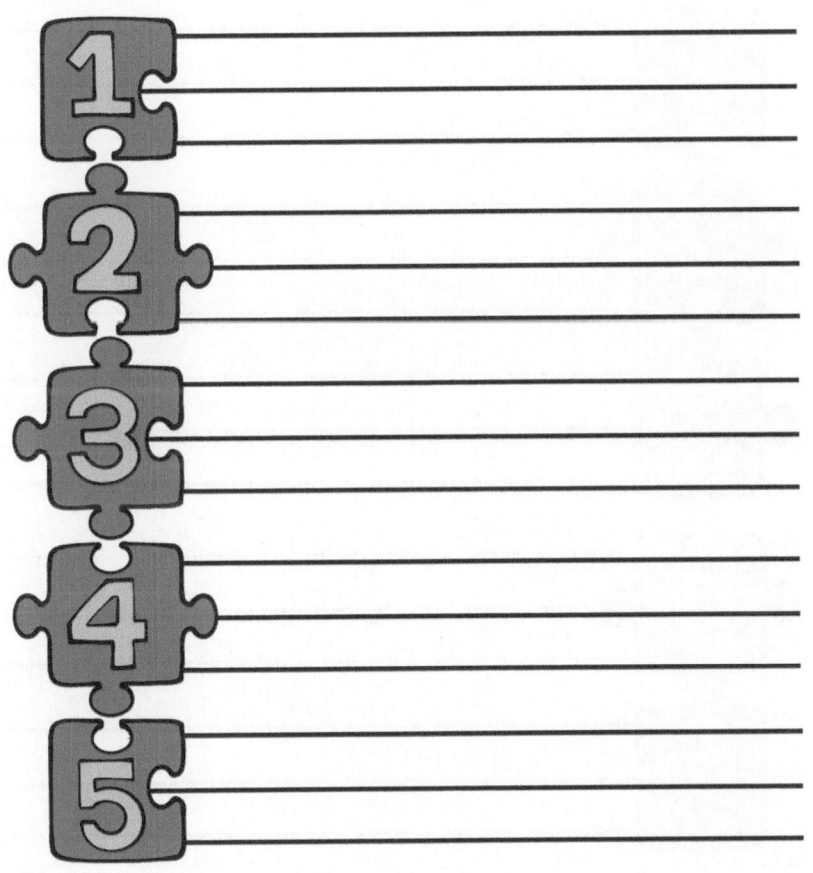

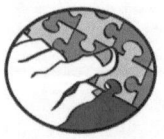

BEHAVIORAL ACTIVATION: PRESCRIPTION PILLS AND OTHER SUBSTANCES MISUSE

The development of a positive behavioral activation plan can help achieve a targeted goal, hopefully leading to improved mood and increased physical wellness. The goal to increase the confidence about changing the behavior of prescription pill and other substance misuse can be broken down into smaller bite-sized objectives. List three to five options one could take to reduce prescription pill misuse or any other identified substance that is being abused.

Goal: Reduce prescription pills and other substances misuse

Behavioral Activation Plan: List three to five ways to reduce prescription pill or other substance misuse

---

Resource Box

- Find treatment at the Substance Abuse and Mental Health Services Administration's website
- Search Web MD's website for information on addictions such as prescription drug abuse

---

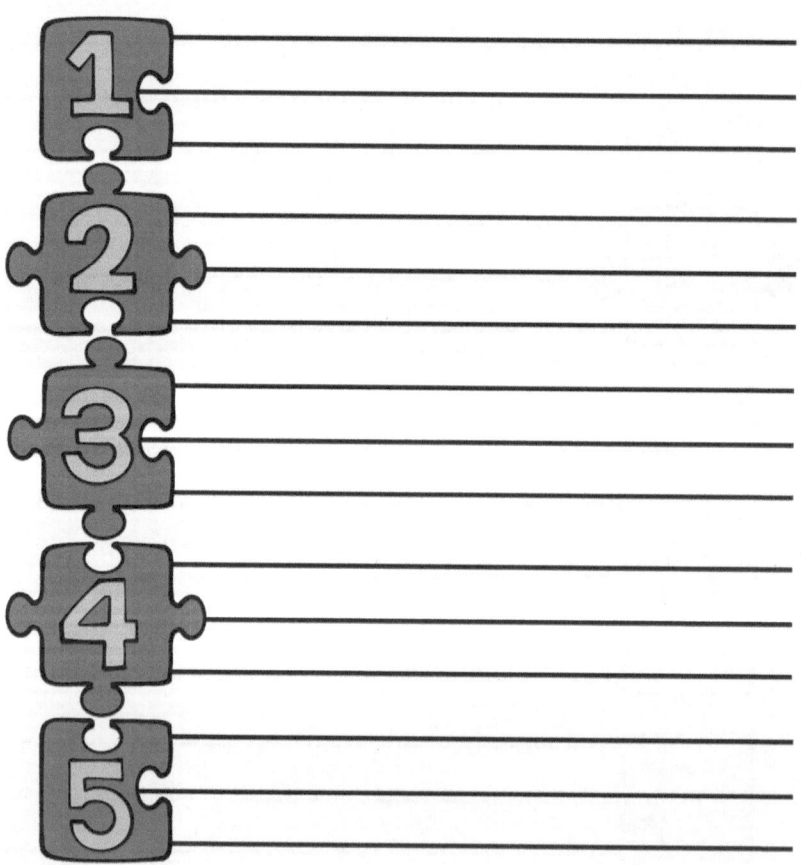

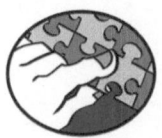

BEHAVIORAL ACTIVATION: NICOTINE AND MARIJUANA MISUSE

The development of a positive behavioral activation plan can help achieve a targeted goal, hopefully leading to improved mood and increased physical wellness. The goal is to increase the confidence about changing the behavior of nicotine or marijuana misuse. List three to five options one could take to reduce nicotine or marijuana misuse.

Goal: Reduce nicotine or marijuana misuse

Behavioral Activation Plan: List three to five ways to reduce nicotine or marijuana misuse

---

Resource Box

- Get tools, tips, and resources from the United States Government's website Smoke Free
- Find support and fellowship on the Marijuana Anonymous website

---

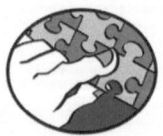

BEHAVIORAL ACTIVATION: ALCOHOL MISUSE

The development of a positive behavioral activation plan can help achieve a targeted goal, hopefully leading to improved mood and increased physical wellness. The goal is to increase the confidence about changing the behavior of alcohol misuse. List three to five options one could take to reduce alcohol misuse.

Goal: Reduce alcohol misuse

Behavioral Activation Plan: List three to five ways to reduce alcohol misuse

---

Resource Box

- Find support and fellowship on the Alcoholics Anonymous website
- Psychoeducational publications can be found on the National Institute on Alcohol Abuse and Alcoholism

---

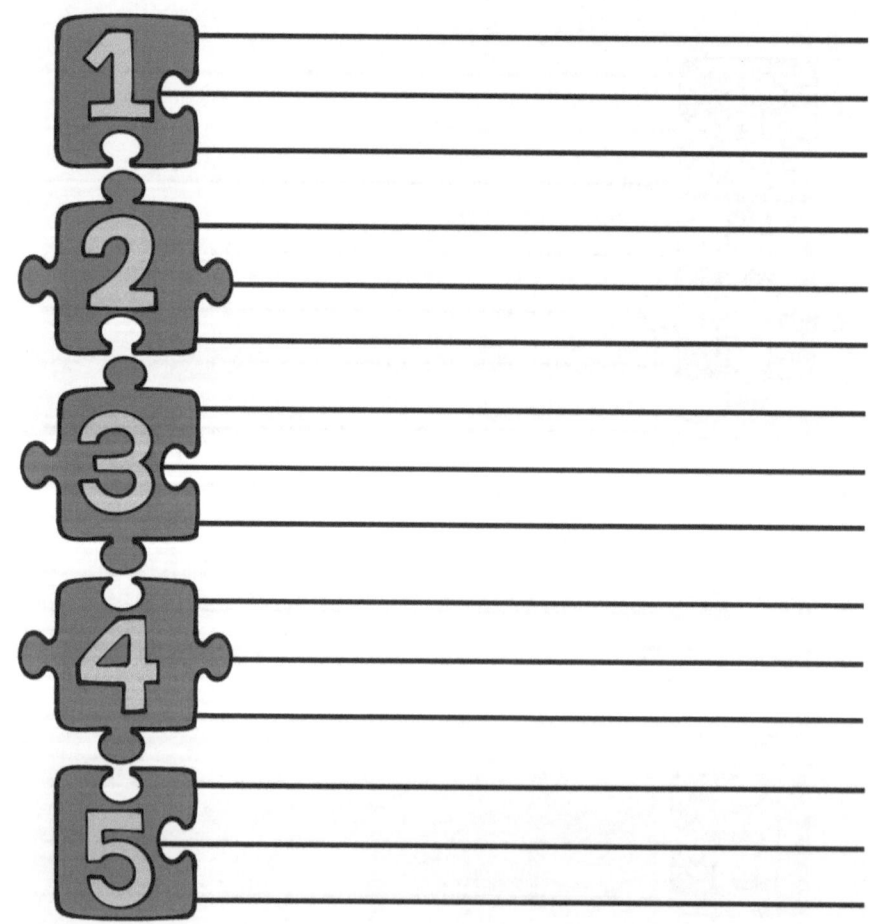

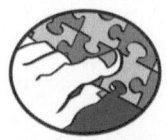

BEHAVIORAL ACTIVATION: INTIMATE PARTNER RELATIONAL PROBLEMS

Developing a positive behavioral activation plan can help achieve a targeted goal, hopefully leading to improved mood, behavior, and communication patterns. The goal is to increase the confidence about changing the behavior causing the problems. List three to five options one could take to reduce intimate partner relational problems.

Goal: Reduce intimate partner relational problems

Behavioral Activation Plan: List three to five ways to reduce intimate partner relational problems

---

Resource Box

- Find a couple therapist on the International Centre for Excellent in Emotionally Focused Therapy website
- Search for intimate partner violence resources on the website for the Centers for Disease Control and Prevention

---

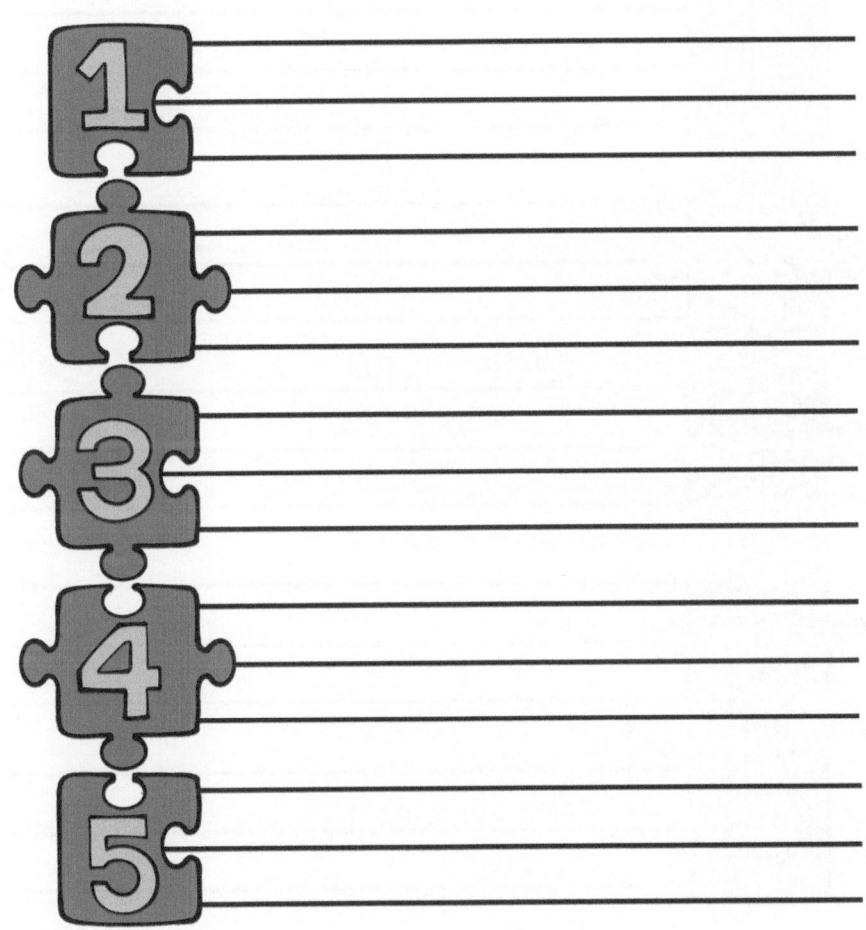

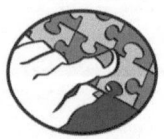

BEHAVIORAL ACTIVATION: SLEEP HYGIENE

The development of a positive behavioral activation plan can help achieve a targeted goal, hopefully leading to improved mood and increased physical wellness. The goal is to increase the confidence about changing the behavior of your sleep hygiene. List three to five options one could take to improve sleep hygiene.

Goal: Improve sleep hygiene

Behavioral Activation Plan: List three to five ways to improve sleep hygiene

---

Resource Box

- Visit the Harvard Medical School webpage on healthy sleep
- The Calm app is a paid resource for meditation and sleep
- Search for sleep hygiene resources on the website for the Centers for Disease Control and Prevention

---

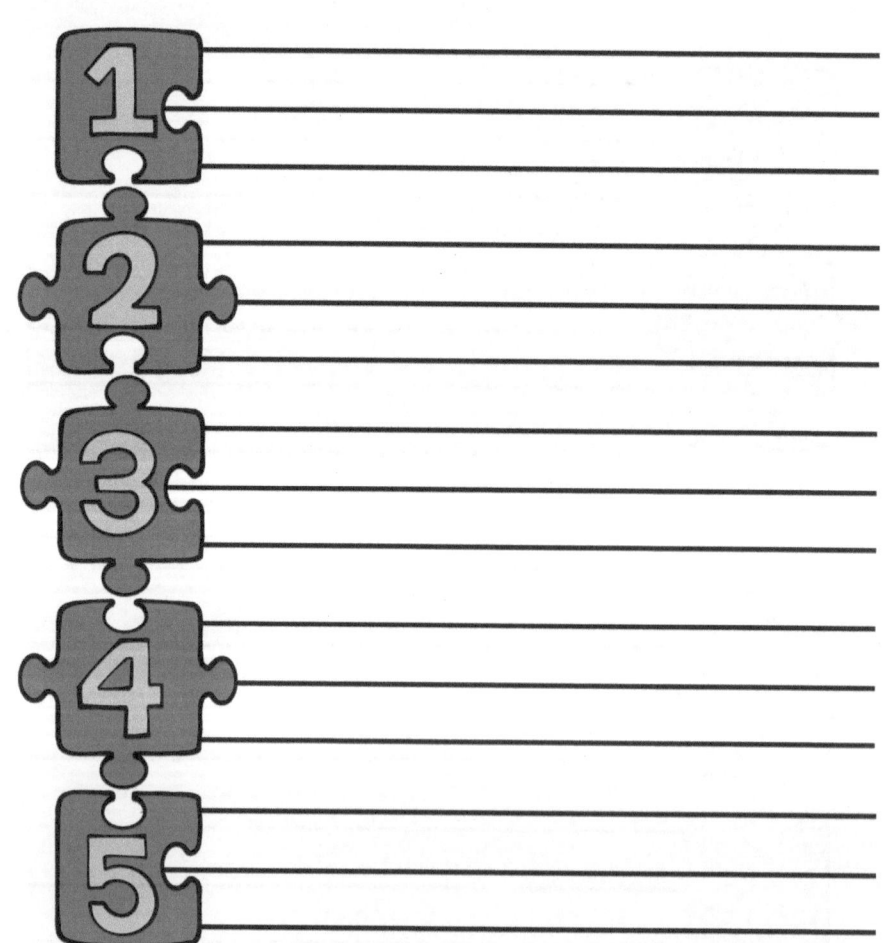

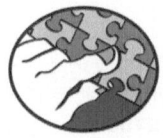 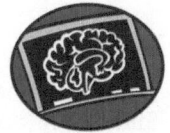

BEHAVIORAL ACTIVATION: DAILY NUTRITION PUZZLE

This infographic shows where one can obtain all of one's daily vitamins. Cut out the nutrition puzzle pieces and use them as behavioral trackers to monitor your daily vitamin intake (suggestions not vegan, not dairy-free or seed/nut-free, but are gluten-free). Be mindful of dietary restrictions and allergies when using this creative nutritional monitoring tool. Remember to drink water (for an average adult daily): 11–15 cups or 2.7–3.7 liters (CDC, 2016).

Goal: Eat well-balanced meals daily, and maintain hydration, making sure to take in the personally appropriate amount of daily vitamins

---

Resource Box

- Visit the Wed MD website and search psychoeducation on vitamins and minerals
- Search for information on the best foods for vitamins and minerals on the staying healthy section of the Harvard Health Publishing at the Harvard Medical School website
- Diet and nutrition support on the Noom paid website with a CBT focus

---

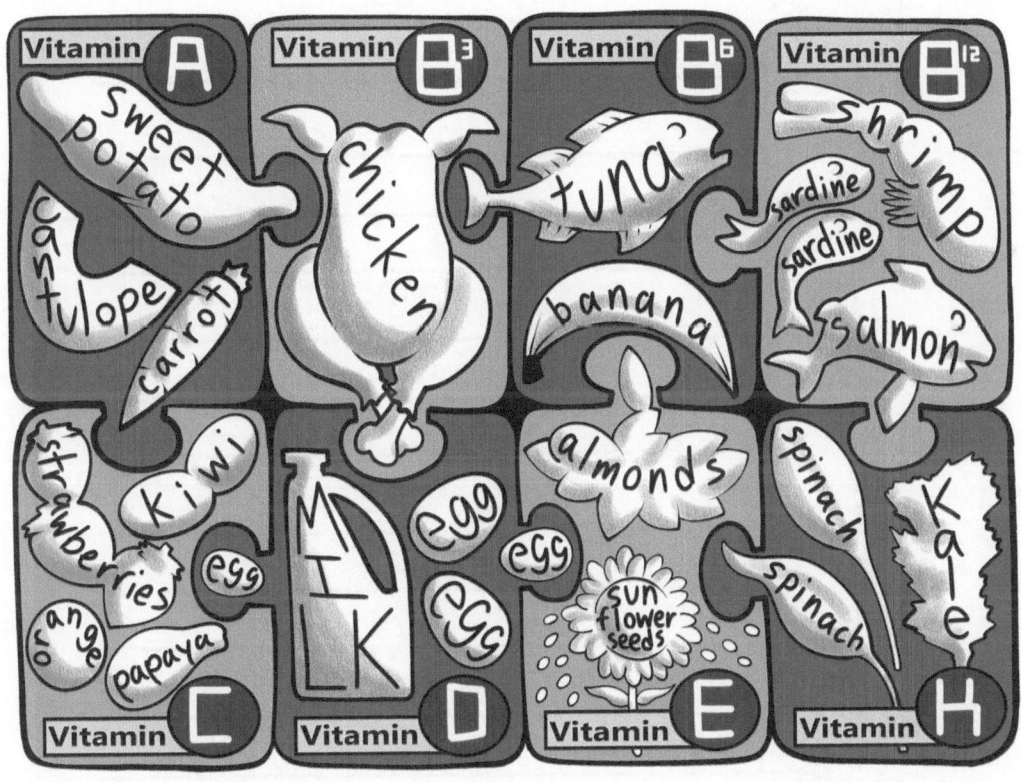

Sample Menu

Breakfast	• Eggs (Vitamin D) • Bell Pepper (Vitamin C, K1) • Onion (Vitamin C) • Canadian Bacon (Vitamin B6) or Vegan breakfast option • Fruit smoothie with fruit listed in the puzzle, protein powder, and milk of choice	Snack	• Cantaloupe (Vitamin A) • Bananas (Vitamin B6) • Strawberries (Vitamin C) • Kiwi (Vitamin C) • Orange (Vitamin C) • Papaya (Vitamin C)
Snack	• Seeds – Sunflower (Vitamin E) • Nuts – Almonds (Vitamin E)	Dinner	• Spinach (Vitamin K) • Sweet Potatoes (Vitamin A) • Salmon or Shrimp (Vitamin B12)
Lunch	• Baby Kale (Vitamin K) • Oil & Vinegar (Vitamin E, K) • Herb-Seasoned Chicken (Vitamin B3)		

Additional disclaimer: While author and illustrator attended USC and UCLA, neither is a nutritionist or dietician, nor are we providing medical advice; this infographic is a creative way to visualize what one might eat to get all of the recommended daily allowances for vitamins in a healthy and fresh manner.

Behavioral Activation Plan: List three to five ways to improve eating well-balanced meals and snacks and ways to improve hydration behaviors

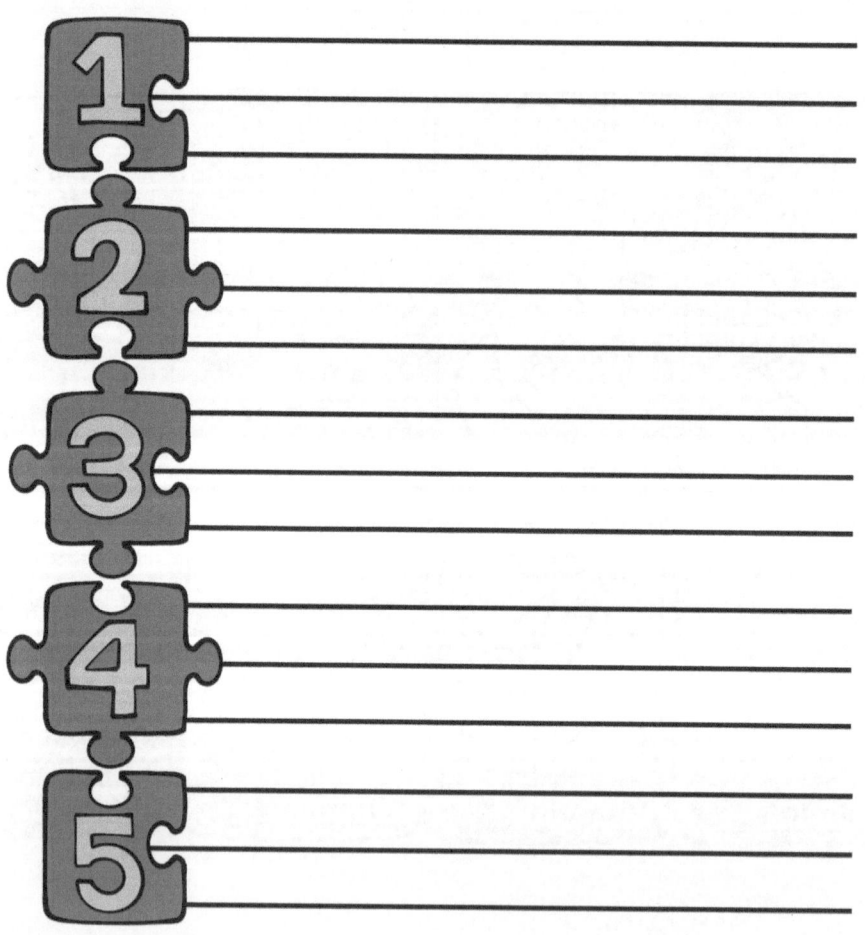

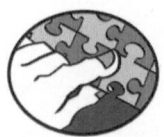

BEHAVIORAL ACTIVATION: EXERCISE ROUTINE

Increasing one's physical activity through cardiovascular exercise will generally improve both mental and physical health. Developing a positive behavioral activation plan can help achieve a targeted goal, hopefully leading to improved mood. The goal is to increase the confidence about changing the behavior of your exercise routine. List three to five options one could take to improve their exercise routine. Daily exercising has been found to be effective in disease prevention and improved mood.

Goal: Improve exercise routine

Behavioral Activation Plan: List three to five ways to improve your exercise routine

---

Resource Box

- At the Self website discover health, fitness, food resources and more
- *Men's Health* magazine is a glossy resource in print and on the web

---

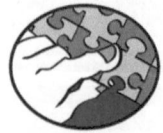 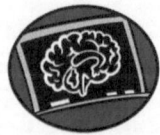

BREAST CANCER SELF-ASSESSMENT

The Breast Cancer Screening handout was inspired by the advocacy of a social work graduate student intern from the Los Angeles LGBT Center. The project was funded by the California State Department of Health Care Services to increase breast cancer awareness for sexual minority women. The project was designed as a psychoeducational tool that engages stakeholders' by utilizing art to support breast cancer education and screening in the LBTQI community. The original artwork is from artist and activist Patricia Bonilla (1998).

Understanding, acknowledging, and validating the following for many lesbians, bisexual women, trans men, and queer and intersex people from the LBTQI community is core to becoming a competent LBTQI affirming therapist, while at the same time considering the intersectionality of sex, assigned sex at birth (ASAB), gender, sexual identity (orientation), skin color, ethnicity, and culture:

- Homophobia, misogyny, transphobia, and racism may lower breast cancer screening rates;
- Lesbians, bisexual women, trans men, and queer and intersex people may be perceived at lower risk for breast cancer;
- Negative experience with past medical doctors or providers may impact current motivation to seek screening and prevention services or treatment;
- General mistrust of the medical community due to personal or historical trauma and/or homophobia, transphobia, and/or misogamy;
- Fears of discrimination;
- Lower rates of health insurance;
- For more information visit the Cancer.org website.

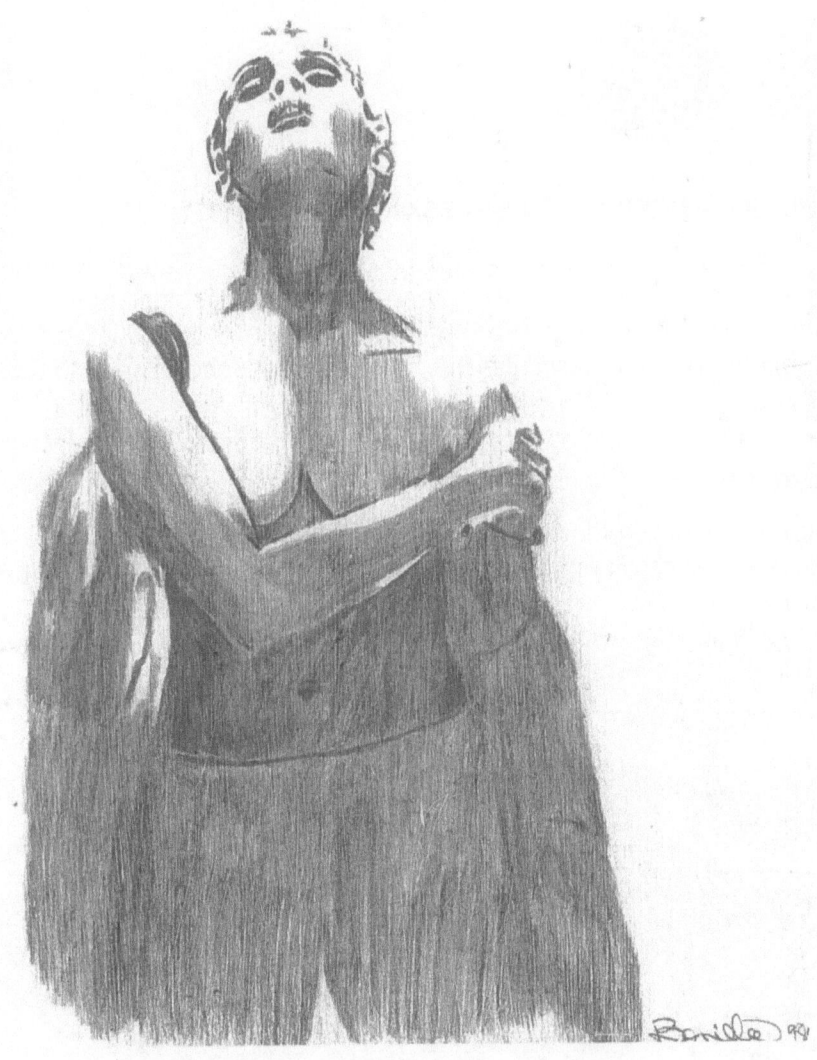

Resource Box

- Information on conducting a breast self-exam can be found at Breastcancer. org
- Search for breast cancer resources on the website for the Centers for Disease Control and Prevention
- Psychoeducational tools and resources are available on the Susan G. Komen breast cancer website
- Visit the Johns Hopkins Medicine website and search the Breast Center in Baltimore, Maryland for resources

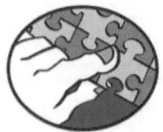 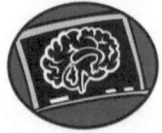

TESTICULAR CANCER SELF-ASSESSMENT

This handout was inspired by the prior on increasing breast cancer awareness. It was designed as a psychoeducational tool that engages stakeholders' by utilizing art to support testicular cancer education and screening in the GBTQI community. The compelling artwork is title *Testicular Cancer* from artist Spencer Afonso (2019).

> **Resource Box**
>
> - Information on conducting a testicular self-exam can be found at the Testicular Cancer Foundation website and also at the Testicular Cancer Society
> - Find social services resources on the Testicular Cancer Awareness Foundation website

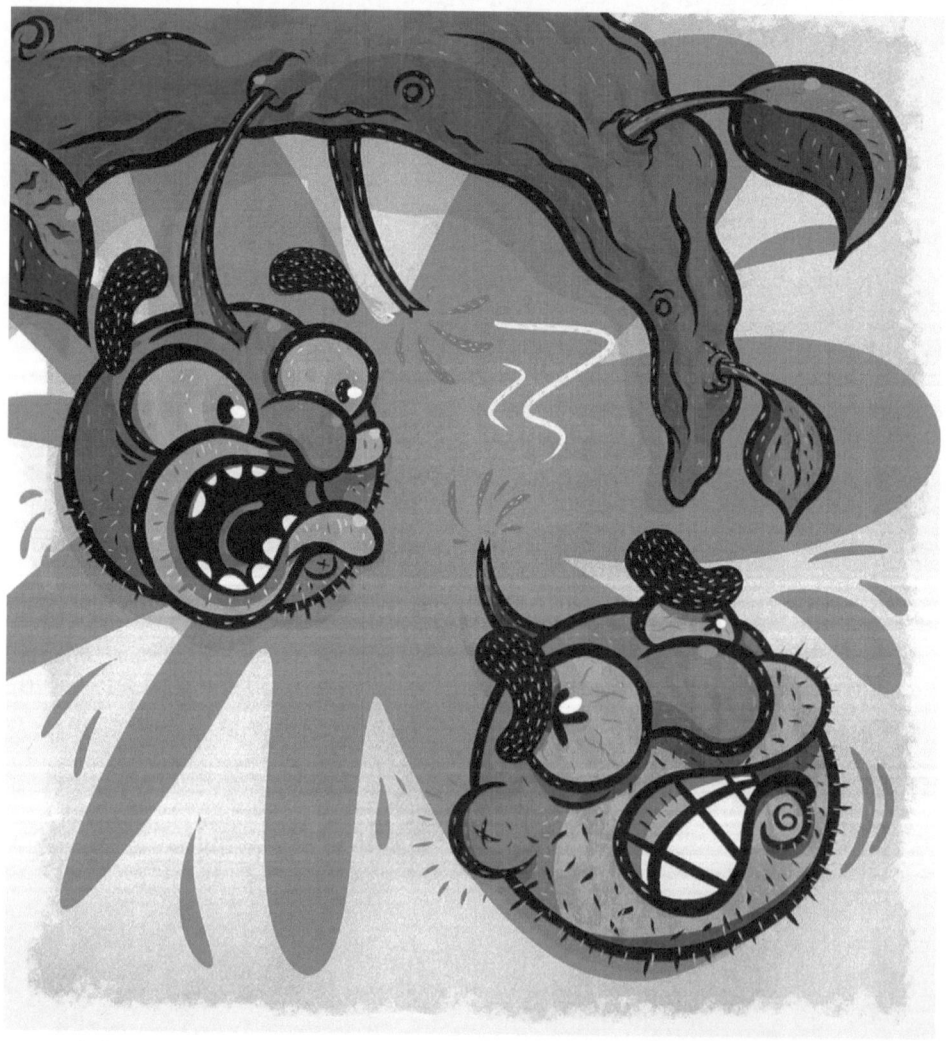

Similar to the breast cancer awareness handout, understanding, acknowledging, and validating the following for many gay and bisexual men, trans women, and queer and intersex people from the GBTQI community is core to becoming a competent GBTQI affirming therapist, while at the same time considering the intersectionality of sex, assigned sex at birth (ASAB), gender, sexual identity (orientation), skin color, ethnicity, and culture:

- Homophobia, misogyny, transphobia, and racism may lower testicular cancer screening rates;
- Gay and bisexual men, trans women, and queer and intersex people may be perceived at lower risk for testicular cancer;
- Caucasians are at higher risk than other ethic identities;
- An undescended testicle is one of the biggest risk-factors;
- Personal or family history of testicular cancer increases risk;
- Living with HIV/AIDS is a risk factor for this type of cancer;
- Negative experience with past medical doctors or providers may impact current motivation to seek screening and prevention services or treatment;
- General mistrust of the medical community due to personal or historical trauma and/or homophobia, transphobia, and/or misogamy;
- Fears of discrimination;
- Lower rates of health insurance;
- For more information visit the Cancer.org website.

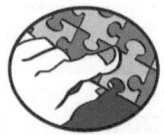

GROUNDING TECHNIQUES 101

Grounding Techniques are relevant and helpful techniques to be included in one's psychological toolbox. These are tools used to assist one in staying in the present moment during episodes of anxiety or panic. One can't change the past, and one has no control over the future. Staying in the present moment is all one can do, which can allow one to feel safe and in control. This is done by focusing on the physical world and how one experiences it in any given moment in time. For the LGBTQI community, each person has experienced trauma that is deeply personal. Create an individual grounding technique that reflects who one is (suggestions are given below).

Grounding is easy to do, and one begins by bringing focus on some aspect of the physical world, like staring at a tree or photo, rather than ruminating on your internal thoughts and feelings. Focus on the present, not the past. Homework is essential for practicing so that one begins to activate a grounding technique automatically when one is triggered.

Here are some suggestions for grounding techniques (or make one up):

- Run cool or warm water over hands;
- Clench chair as hard as you can;
- Touch various things around oneself;
- Literally ground oneself by pushing feet onto the floor with all edges of the foot touching the ground;
- Lay directly on the ground or floor;
- Carry a grounding object with you like a stone in your pocket, and touch it when feeling triggered;
- Use an app on your smartphone or watch to help guide relaxation;
- Notice your body: pay attention to the weight in the chair, wiggle your toes, roll your feet out, and stretch and massage each finger individually;
- Stretch, and do neck rolls;
- Clench fists, then release, and repeat for one minute;
- Do mindful walking, very slowly, where one notices each footstep;
- Do deep breathing (see Bunny Breath handout);
- Eat some nuts or dried fruit, describing the experience based on one's five senses (taste, sight, touch, smell, and sound);
- Calm Place, Bunny Breath, Mini-Sandtray, Body Scan, and Hero Coloring handouts and worksheets are all viable grounding techniques depending on one's interest.

Resource Box

- Master the practice of mindfulness at the Headspace paid website
- Learn meditation on the Ten Percent Happier paid website
- Track mood and find support on the Mood Panda web and mobile app

---

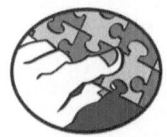 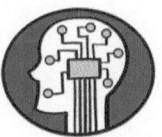

GROUNDING TECHNIQUE: CALM PLACE

This technique will take you through your five senses (taste, sight, touch, smell, and sound) to help remind you of the present. This is a calming technique that can help you get through tough or stressful situations. This tool is also important when doing trauma work using the Eye Movement Desensitization and Reprocessing (EMDR) intervention. Establishing a protective grounding technique is essential before beginning any intensive trauma-focused psychotherapy or for everyday use when stress symptoms are present (Shapiro, 2017).

Directions: First, select an image for your calm place – a beach, your bed, a space where you can feel safe, or at least at best feel calm.

Take a deep belly breath or use the Bunny Breath technique to begin. Begin to activate your five senses based on your image selected.

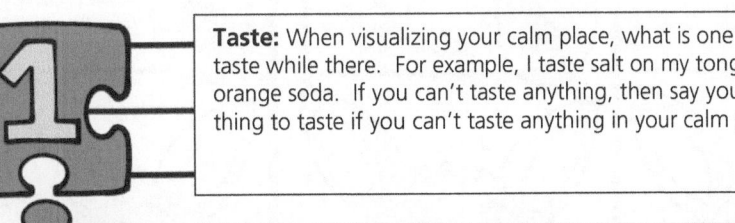

Taste: When visualizing your calm place, what is one thing you taste while there. For example, I taste salt on my tongue, or I taste orange soda. If you can't taste anything, then say your favorite thing to taste if you can't taste anything in your calm place.

Smell: Identify at least 2 things you can smell while visualizing your calm place. For example, I smell salt in the crisp beach air, or I smell coconut fragrance from suntan lotion . If you can't smell anything at the moment, maybe think about a smell you might like to now associate with this calm place image, like lavender or citrus.

Listen/Auditory: Listen for at least 3 sounds in your clam place. For example, it could be the wind in the trees, the crashing of the waves, or the birds overhead.

Feel/Touch: Direct your awareness internally and think of 4 things that you can feel. For example, at the beach, you could say, I feel my feet warming in the sand, then coolingin the water, I feel the wind in my hair, I feel supported and grounded sitting in the sand on a soft blanket.

Look/Sight: Look around your calm place and identify at least 5 things that you can see and describe all the colors that are present. For example, a calm place could be the coves at Leo Carrillo State Beach in Malibu, California, you could say, I see the turquoise sea, the white caps on the waves, the creamy light brown sand, yellow sun, green and brown palm trees, pink and purple sun umbrellas, and red life-guard station.

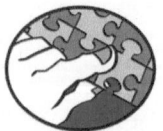

GROUNDING TECHNIQUE: BUNNY BREATH

Alternate nostril breathing is an ancient yoga grounding technique. *Nadi shodhana pranayama* is the Sanskrit word for alternate nostril breathing, or *Bunny Breath*, translating to *a subtle energy clearing breathing technique*. This type of breathwork can be done as part of a yoga or meditation practice or in trauma work. Alternate nostril breathing can also be done as its own practice to help quiet and still one's mind before bed or a test.

Directions: Follow the instructions in the infographic to increase oxygen flow to the brain and expand the lungs in order to promote relaxation and decrease anxiety and stress.

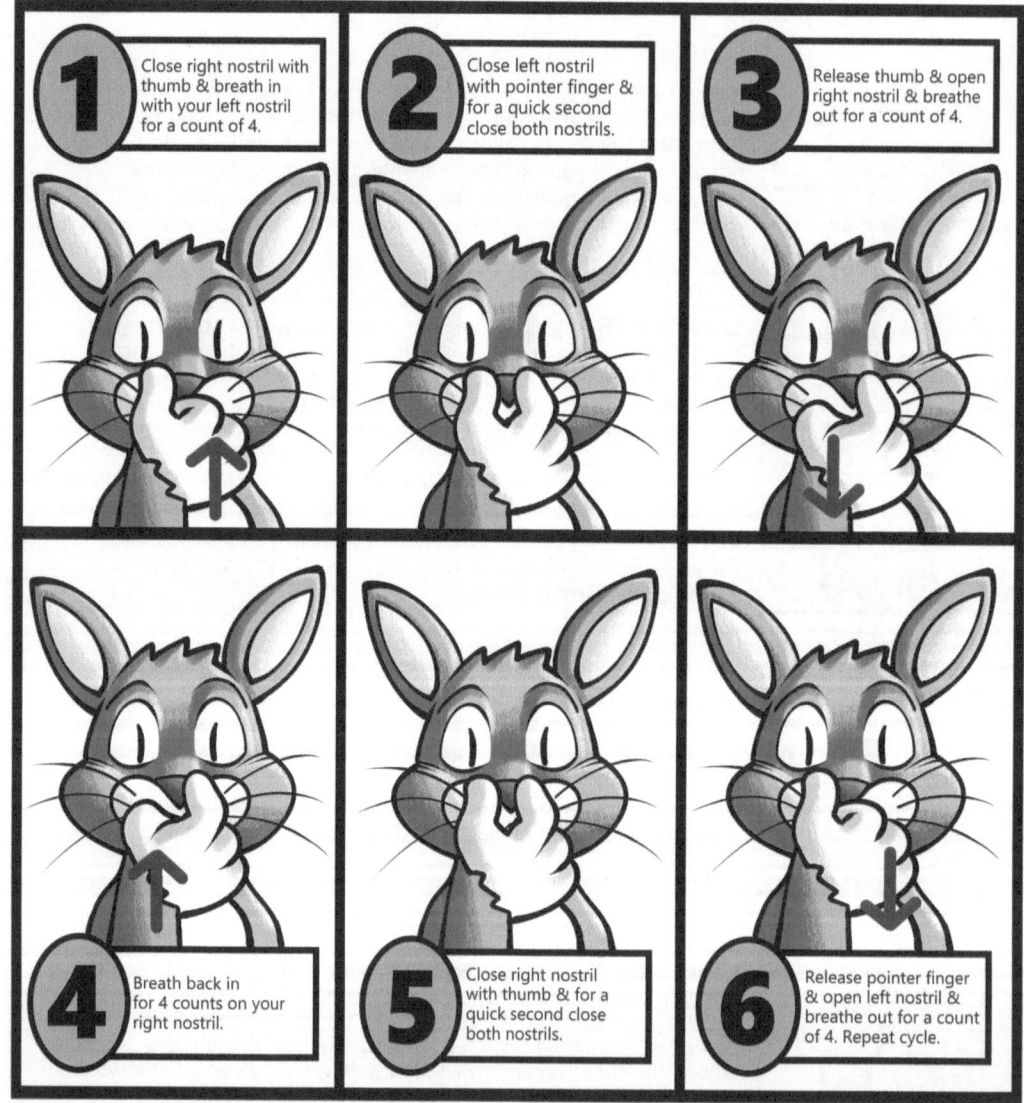

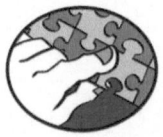 

GROUNDING TECHNIQUE: MINI-SANDTRAY

Sandtray Therapy (ST) for adults and couples is a popular therapeutic technique. For more on ST, check out a video created by Dr. Schott and Sandtray Therapy expert Dr. Helen Land, LCSW which can be found on YouTube.

Sandtray Therapy helps bring the brain online in ways that traditional talk therapies might miss. Not everyone expresses their trauma through talk therapy; sometimes, therapies are expressive, like dance or art therapy. Trauma in the LGBTQI community is unfortunately pervasive, and enacting an expression of healing through miniatures using the sandtray technique can be a powerful clinical tool. Running your hands through the sand is a grounding technique, similar to the Clam Place handout.

Directions: Materials needed to make your mini-sandtray (author's sandtray is an example in the photo):

1. Storage container that seals (~11″ × 8″ × 3″ is ideal or any size you desire really). If you get a container with the bottom colored in blue, then skip step 2. Blue represents water in the sandtray technique.
2. Blue paper and tape or glue. Cut blue paper to fit the bottom of the container, and then tape or glue it in place.
3. Sand (fine textured sand has been shown to be most effective). Fill your tray (~8 cups or to your desire).
4. Tools. To manipulate sand, like a miniature rake or a small spoon or fork, etc.
5. Miniatures. They can be mini cars; fast food meal gifts; mini people; animals; building blocks; mini toys; fake or dried vegetation; fences; mini signs; natural items you find, like rocks or dried flowers; fantasy items; action figures; spiritual minis, like crosses or Buddha; gemstones; religious symbols; and household (old salt and pepper shaker) or medical mini objects.

Author's favorite sandtray self-reflection activity: Divide empty sandtray into three sections, select miniatures to represent the past life (left of tray), present life (middle of tray), and future life template (right side of tray). Arrange miniatures into sandtray that represent these three domains in one's life and reflect on past, present, and future self-identity and goals.

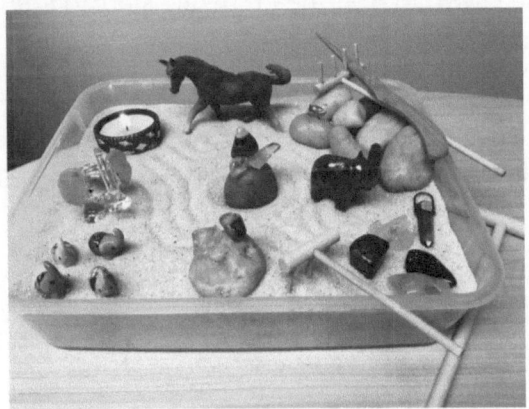

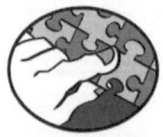

GROUNDING TECHNIQUE: BODY SCAN

The body scan grounding technique is a powerful clinical tool rooted in the evidence-based practice of Mindfulness Based-Stress Reduction (MBSR). The body scan's purpose is to help you tune in to your body and reconnect to your physical self. The goal is to notice any sensations you're feeling without judgment. Relaxation can be a result of performing this technique, but it is not the primary goal. The goal is to train the mind to be more open and aware of sensory experiences. Ultimately, this creates more self-acceptance. With time and practice, the body scan can build your ability to focus and be fully present in your daily life (Dreeben, Mamberg, & Salmon, 2013).

Our Reptile Brain ignites the *flight* or *fight* response when a trigger occurs, and we get stuck due to our LGBTQI traumas (refer to Your LGBTQI Brain handout). The Limbic System and Neocortex are the brain regions one hopes to return to after invoking grounding techniques.

Resource Box

- Take a 45-minute body scan guided meditation from the University of California at San Diego Center for Mindfulness, which is used as part of training for the Mindfulness-Based Stress Reduction (MBSR) intervention
- Practice a body scan meditation from the Greater Good in Action website at the University of California at Berkeley
- Take mindfulness courses on the Mindful USC website at the University of Southern California
- Mindful Awareness Research Center (MARC) on the University of California at Los Angeles Health website host classes and events on mindfulness practice

---

Directions: Quick Three-Minute Seven-Step Body Scan:

1. Sit comfortably and close your eyes;
2. Take a deep breath in through the nose, and out through the mouth;
3. Notice how your entire body feels right now;
4. Beginning at the crown of your head, gently start to scan down through your entire body;
5. Notice what feels comfortable and what feels uncomfortable;
6. The goal is not trying to change anything, just noticing how the body feels as you scan down evenly;
7. Notice each and every part of the body, all the way down to your toes.

CBT/ABC Physiology Body Scan

Directions: In the boxes, begin by recording the activating event, then record your cognitions, emotions, and behaviors that followed. Using the Identity Iguana graphic as a personal physiological map, write down next to the appropriate arrow any physical reactions, feelings, or sensations you are experiencing which corresponds to the respective body part on the Iguana image. These physiological reactions can be in response to one's cognitions, emotions, and behaviors in the CBT model.

Trigger or Activation (A):

Cognitions (C) or Beliefs (B):

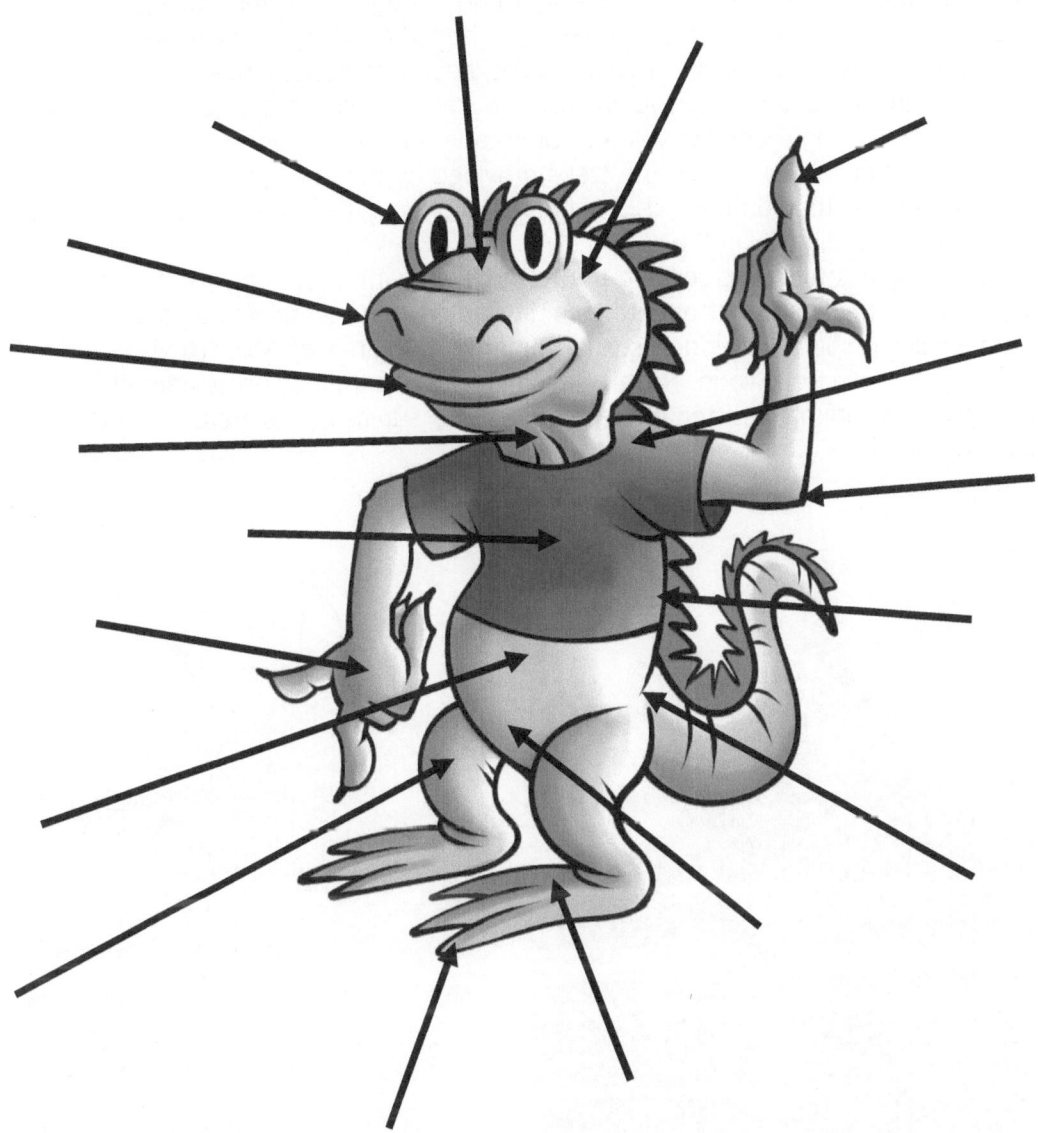

Emotions:

Behavior (B) or Consequence (C):

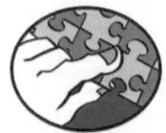 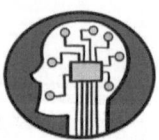

GROUNDING TECHNIQUE: HERO MINDFUL COLORING ACTIVITY

Adult coloring has beneficial impacts on mental health (Fitzpatrick, 2017). For the LGBTQI community, this is especially important to note as individuals may find expression through art can often be a very personally cathartic experience. Many from the LGBTQI community lack the visual presence of positive role models. This activity hopes to create a positive visualization.

Directions: Think about your hero that you would like to color. Select a favorite image or photo of a hero you admire and find strength in. Alternatively, you could select a photo of a beloved pet that has brought you comfort. You will need a printer and paper, along with crayons, pencils, paint, and/or markers. Once you gather your materials and select a photo, you will use the free Colorscape app to turn the photo into a coloring worksheet. Download Colorscape onto your favorite electronic device (smartphone or tablet). Follow the steps provided by the app, convert the file into a coloring outline, then print it out, and finish by coloring it all in. Alternatively, you can color the photo digitally in the app.

An example could be to select a photo of Cary Grant, assuming you find strength in the actor. The legendary "queer" actor struggled with mental health issues and the complexities of being a hidden sexual minority in a time of McCarthyism and the Lavender Scare in Hollywood. The example below is of a therapy horse named Gerome that provided animal assisted therapy to trauma survivors – a hero to many who worked with him.

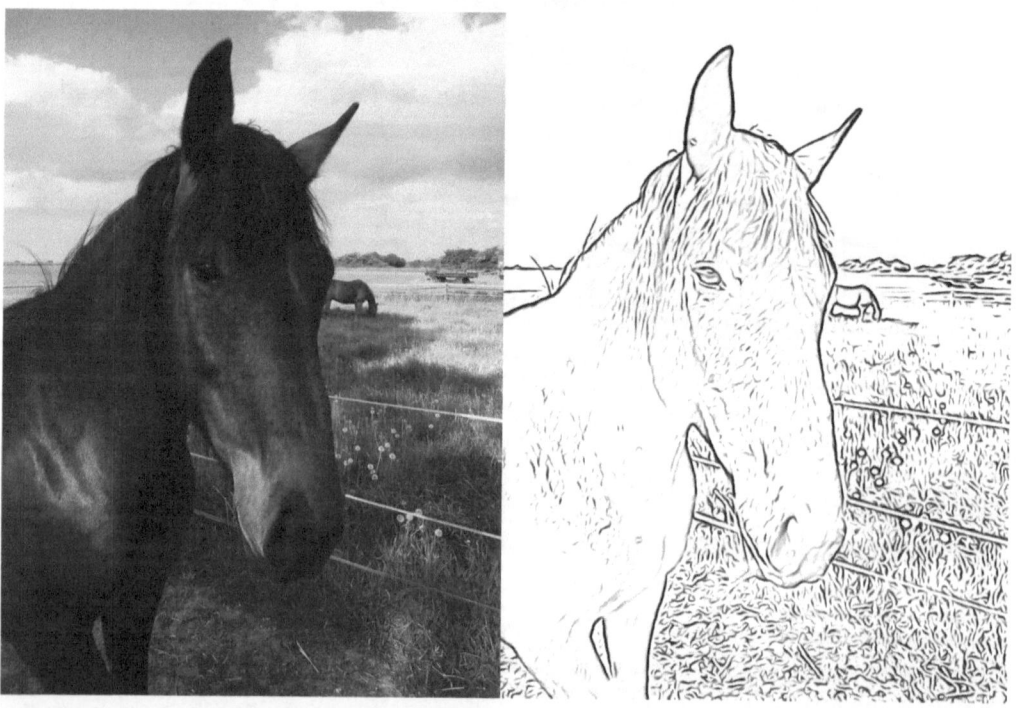

Part 4

Psychoeducational Handouts and Worksheets

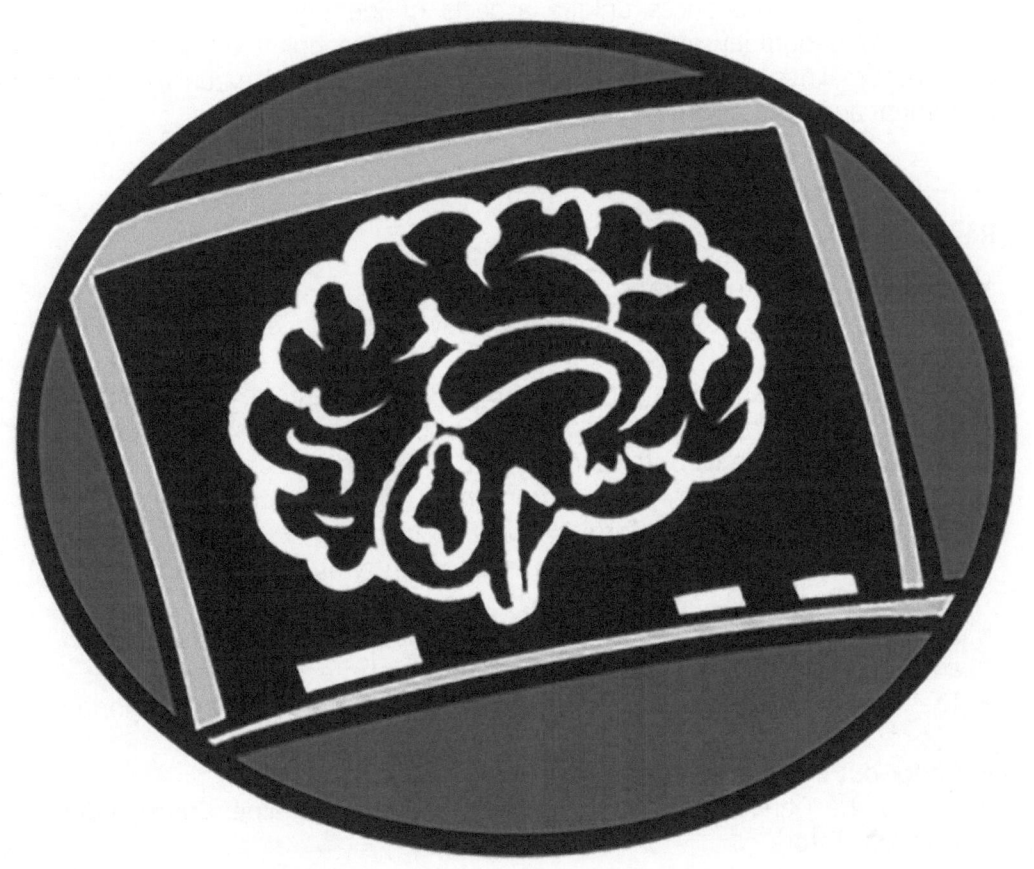

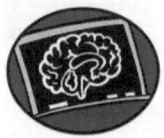

LGBTQI HISTORY

Therapists and clients alike must understand the historical context of identifying as LGBTQI. Everyone experiences unique aspects of identity development that are influenced by geography and culture. In the resource box are some compelling educational timelines to use when educating oneself on the contextual experiences of development and oppression for the LGBTQI community.

Resource Box

- Look over OutHistory's Transgender History Timeline
- Search the Milestones in the American Gay Rights Movement on the PBS website
- Investigate CNN's website for their LGBTQ Rights Milestone Fast Facts
- Find resources from California on LGBTQ history for educators, students, and families on the website Teaching LGBTQ History
- Visit the LGBTQ historical timeline from the LGBTQ+ Student Center on the University of Southern California (USC) website
- Explore the largest LGBTQ archives in the country at the ONE Archives at the USC Libraries
- Remember LGBTQI victims of holocaust at the Institute for Visual History and Education at the USC Shoah Foundation website
- The GLSEN website has history resources such as podcast and coloring books
- Check-out the interACT website
- Review the Canadian Broadcasting Corporation's Timeline: Transgender Through History

---

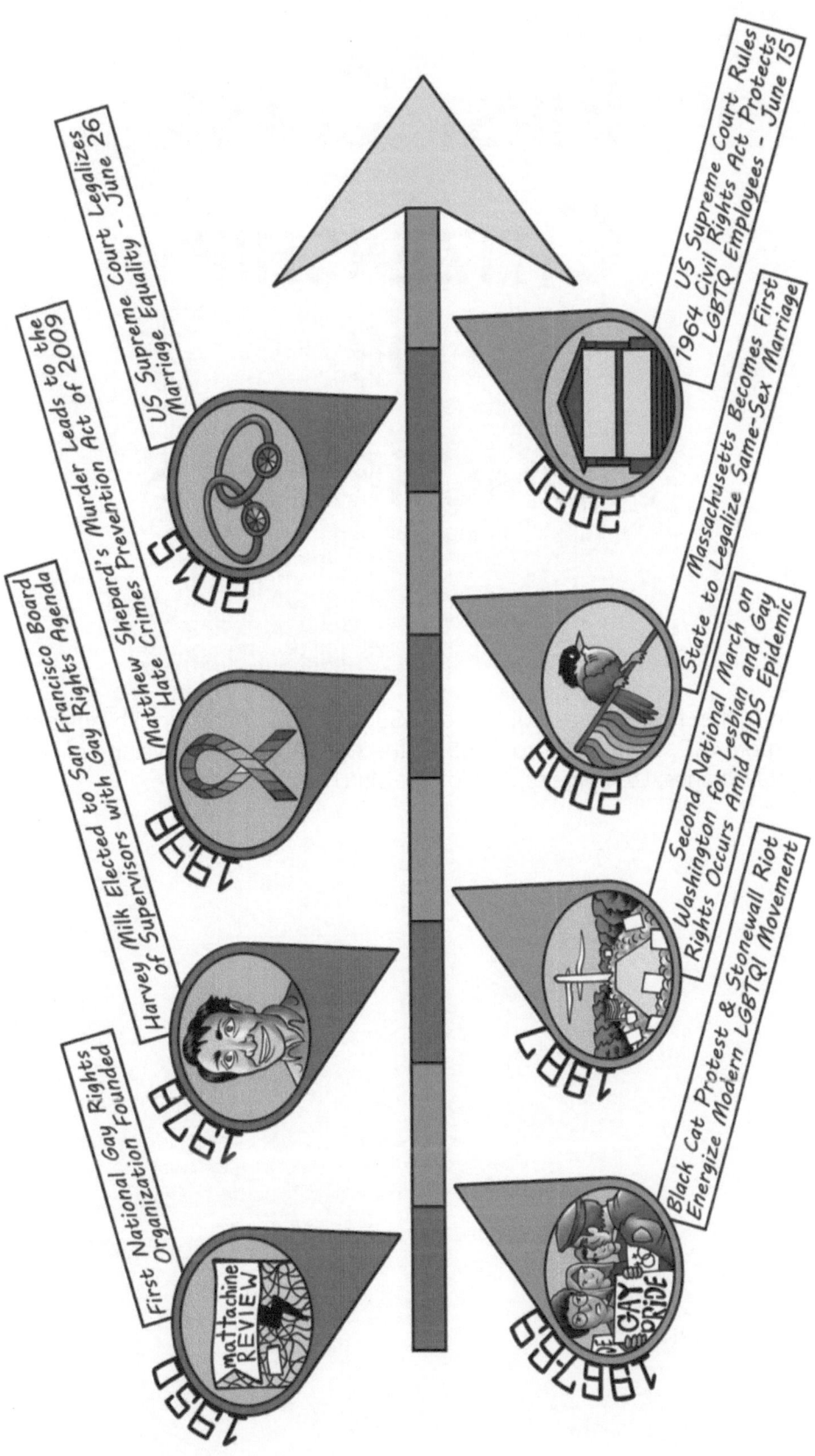

Sign from the first public protest for LGBTQI equal rights in Philadelphia and Washington, D.C. from 1965 to 1969 at the ONE Archives, University of Southern California Libraries, Los Angeles, California. March 29, 2018.

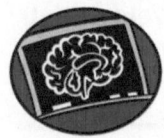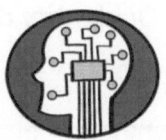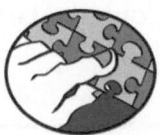

COMING OUT

The coming out developmental journey is different for each LGBTQI individual. Some people may not only hold LGBTQI identities but are also people with differences in abilities, immigrants, and people experiencing a lack of stable affirming housing. Privileges based on holding the dominant narrative are assigned to various identities. The coming-out process can be non-linear and must consider the dynamics of culture and geography. This exercise was designed to be used in conjunction with the Intersectionality Gem handout and worksheet. A variety of experiences and cultural traditions can influence people's understanding of and relationship to LGBTQI identity based on the intersection of their gender identity and racial/ethnic identity. Members of the LGBTQI community hold multiple identities. The community faces multiple oppressions, and considering wellness and safety practices is essential. Creating brave spaces is encouraged. Coming out is personal, and it is about you deciding how, when, and with whom to share your identities.

Resource Box

- Coming out handbook for LGBTQ young people can be found on the Trevor Project website
- GLSEN website has coming out activities and resources for LGBTQ students
- The LGBTQ+ Student Center on the USC website has general tips for coming out
- Human Rights Campaign has searchable resources on their website
- Search the website for the National Center for Transgender Equality
- Discover services and resources on the Los Angeles Gender Center website

---

List five successful steps in your coming out and LGBTQI identity development:

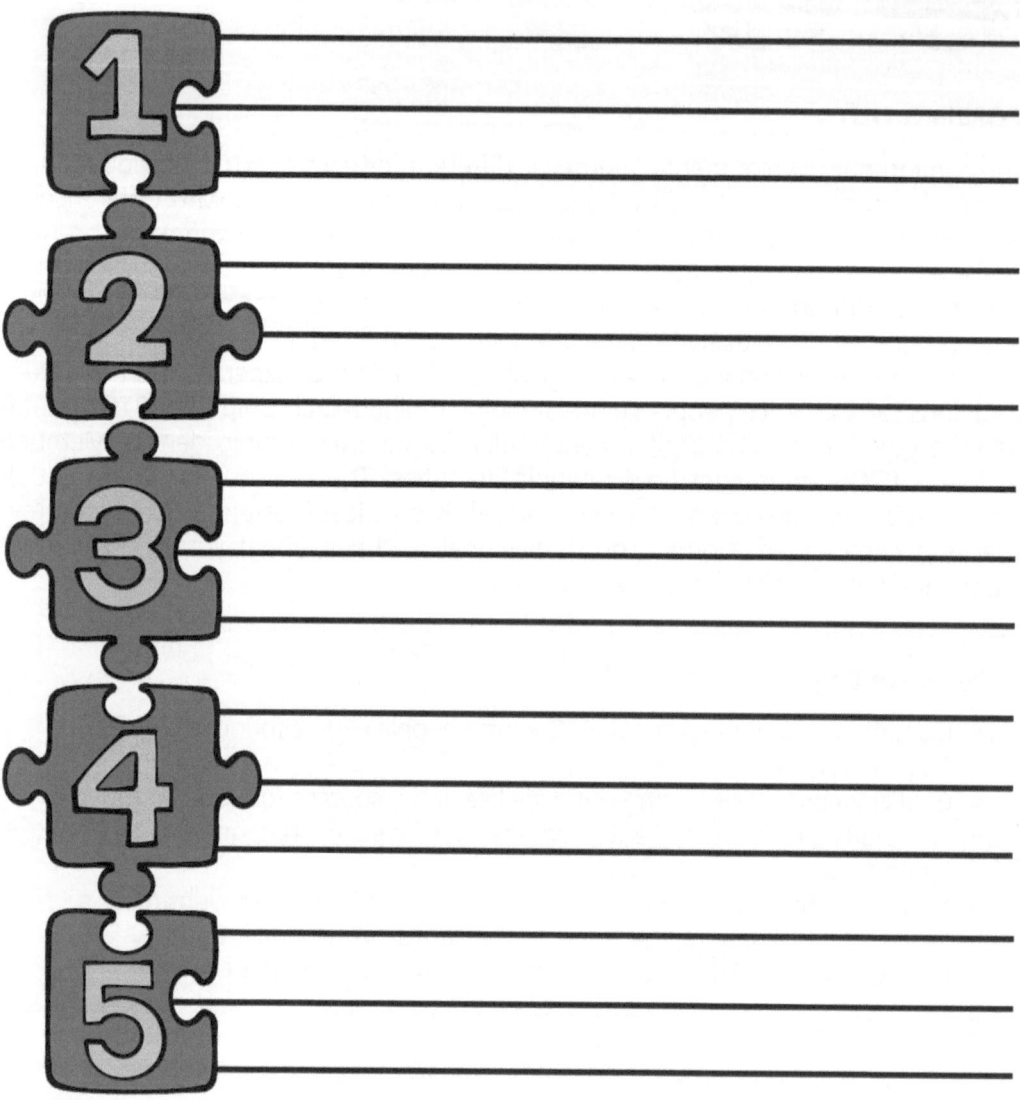

Identify five goals still needing attention to complete your development:

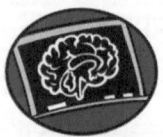

THE LGBTQI IDENTITY IGUANA

The LGBTQI Identity Iguana infographic is a powerful educational tool that helps one understand the concepts of gender identity, sexual identity (orientation), gender expression, sex or assigned sex at birth, physical/romantic/emotional attraction, and the impact of culture and geography.

Gender Identity: One's internal sense of being male, female, both female and male, or neither. All human beings have a gender identity. For transgender people, assigned sex at birth and one's gender identity is incongruent. For cisgender people, assigned sex at birth and one's gender identity is congruent. For intersex people, the term *sex* is generally more inclusive as one's *assigned sex at birth* (ASAB) was often not *intersex*. An intersex person's true sex is *intersex*. The intersex community is often assigned male or female at birth (AMAB or AFAB), causing trauma both psychologically and physically. The individual is left often isolated and invisible.

Gender Expression: Physical manifestation of one's gender identity (clothing, hairstyle, voice, body shape, etc.). Most humans seek to make their gender expression (how they look) match their gender identity (who they are).

Sex or Assigned Sex at Birth: Classification of people as male, female, intersex, or another possibility. Socially assigned based on a combination of anatomy, hormones, and chromosomes.

Physical/Romantic/Emotional Attraction (Sexual Identity [Orientation]): Who one loves.

Culture: One's shared beliefs and customs as a member of a social group.

Geography: One's relationship with physical location.

Directions: Fill in the Identity Iguana with your personal identifiers. Use the chart for examples, but this list is not exhaustive and is ever evolving (go to http://www.silverlakepsychotherapy.com/LGBTQI_identity_iguana for the current version of the infographic in color which can be used as a teaching tool and has permissions granted to be reproduced).

The LGBTQI Identity Iguana

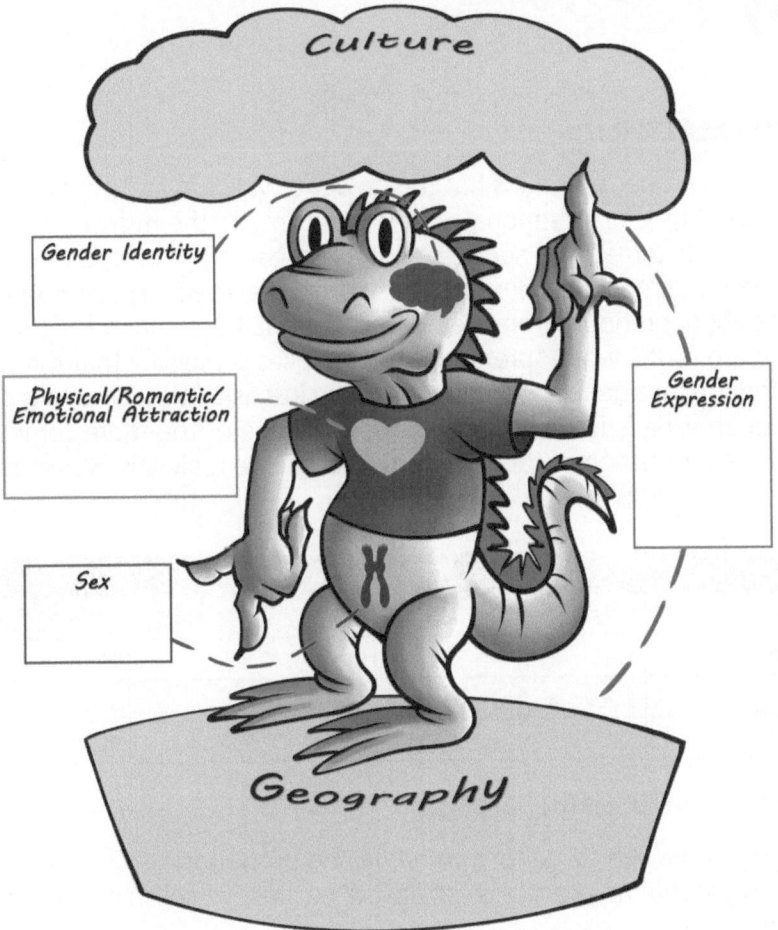

By Erik Schott and Cody Wilson at www.silverlakepsychotherapy.com

Identity Concept:	Gender Identity	Gender Expression	Sex	Physical/ Romantic/ Emotional Attraction	Culture	Geography
Examples of identities:	• Queer • Woman • Irans Man • Trans Woman • Man • Transgender • Non-binary • Agender • Gender-fluid • Androgyne • Cisgender • Genderqueer • Gender Nonconforming (GNC) • Pangender • Two-Spirited • Another possibility: _____	• Feminine • Masculine • Gender-Neutral • Androgynous • Another possibility: _____	• Intersex • Assigned Female at Birth • Assigned Male at Birth • Another possibility: _____	• Bisexual • Gay • Lesbian • Heterosexual • Pansexual • Aromantic • Asexual • Another possibility: _____	• Faith beliefs • Government • Family • Community • Role expectations • Gender role strain • Language • National origin • Ethnicity • Minority stress • Skin color • SES • Another possibility: _____	• Hemisphere • Continent • Country • State • Province • Region • City • Another possibility: _____

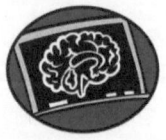

PRONOUNS MATTER

Using a person's proper pronouns has the power to validate and empower. Often the misuse of pronouns is unintentional. In another context, the misuse of pronouns can indicate danger or threat. It is suggested to ask a person what pronouns confirm or go along with ones' gender identity. The word "preferred" is still improperly used when asking about pronouns from members of the LGBTQI community. It is encouraged to avoid the use of the word "preferred" as it implies somehow that there is a choice or another option for a gender identity. One might just ask, "What are your pronouns?"

This is not an exhaustive list of pronouns, but some of the more common ones at the time of the production of this workbook. Language is always evolving, and so the possibility of more pronouns.

Pronouns			
Feminine	She	Her	Hers
Masculine	He	Him	His
Neutral	They	Them	Theirs
Neutral	Ze	Hir/Zir	Hirs/Zirs

Pronoun Inclusion Checklist

- Email signature line contains your name and pronouns
- Don't forget that no pronouns can always be used – English can be written in the passive tense
- Always be mindful that language is ever evolving and there are infinite possibilities regarding the evolution of the use of pronouns
- Inclusive language in literature and text
- Brave or safe physical spaces
- Gender-neutral restrooms
- Visual markers (e.g., pride sticker, pin, or poster/flyer)

Resource Box

- Find resources on the Facebook page for Trans Student Educational Resources
- Uncover education activities at the LGBTQ+ Student Center on the USC website
- Discover on the Anti-Defamation League resources, tools, and strategies for using correct pronouns and names

---

My pronouns are:

Directions: Practice asking a close friend's pronouns. Then in the space below: (1) Describe the interaction, (2) record the emotions experienced, and (3) notice the resonation of any thoughts (cognitions) and/or emotions within one's body as a body scan is conducted.

---

1. **Cognitive (Neocortex):** Description of thoughts of the interaction

2. **Emotional (Limbic System):** Primary emotions experienced during the interaction

3. **Physical/Behavioral:** Body scan with an observation of where the thoughts and emotions are resonating within one's body during the interaction

---

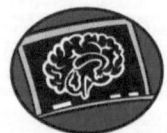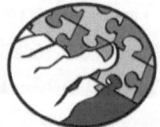

SEXUAL HEALTH CHECKLIST: LBTQI COMMUNITY

This handout was designed as a psychoeducational tool to assist in making decisions related to developing a support around one's sexual health.

Sexual health according to the World Health Organization (Savoy, O' Gurek, & Brown-James, 2020), in relation to human sexuality is a state of physical, mental, and social well-being. Positive sexual health requires a respectful approach to sexuality and sexual relationships. Positive sexual health is free of coercion, discrimination, and violence. Conditions include the possibility of having pleasurable and safe sexual experiences.

Therapists must be comfortable in asking questions and generating a discussion around these issues in order to help clients maintain optimal health.

Following is a sexual health checklist (Poteat, 2012):

1. **Come out to your medical provider**. Your provider needs to know your sexuality because it will help them to order the proper tests and help you maintain optimal health. If you do not feel comfortable talking about these issues with your provider, you can role play this with a therapist or find a provider with whom you feel more comfortable.
2. **Get screened for breast cancer**. More likely to have risk factors for breast cancer and may be less likely to be screened. Discuss this with your doctor regularly, learn how to self-screen. Practice self-screening on a regular basis. Early diagnosis and intervention lead to more successful treatment outcomes.
3. **Get screened for gynecological cancers**. Greater risk for certain types of gynecological cancers than their heterosexual counterparts. Talk with your doctor about these risks and get regular pap smears for early detection and intervention.
4. **Practice safer sex and get the right tests**. Are at risk for the same sexually transmitted infections (STIs) as heterosexual women. If one is sexually active one should be tested regularly for STIs. Talk to your provider about your risk factors. If you are not comfortable speaking with your provider, find one with whom you are comfortable.

   Women are at risk for human papilloma virus (HPV) which can cause genital warts in the vulva or anus areas. Untreated, HPV can lead to various types of cancer. Discuss HPV with your provider. A vaccine can lower your risk of contracting HPV.

   Women are also at risk for gonorrhea, chlamydia, and syphilis. In addition to these more well-known sexually transmitted infections, two additional types of bacteria can be spread between women—vaginosis and trichomoniasis. Oral sex, digital-vaginal, or digital-anal contact can spread any of these infections. These illnesses can also be transmitted through the sharing of sex toys. Sex toys should be washed with warm-soapy water between uses or covered with a new condom with each use.

   Just because you do not notice symptoms of STIs does not mean they are not present. The only way to be certain you are free of infection is to be tested. Without intervention, all of these infections can lead to long-term health consequences. If you believe you are at risk for any of these infections, speak with your provider or go to a local clinic for testing.

While not at high risk for HIV from other women, lesbians, bisexual, and queer women can still be infected if they have a sex partner who is HIV positive. This is especially risky for women who also have sex with men. The safest way to prevent HIV infection is to use condoms if having vaginal, anal, or oral sex with men. Condoms can also prevent pregnancy and other sexually transmitted infections (Poteat, 2012).

Many county funded health providers and clinics also provide free intervention for HIV testing and integrated care. If you believe you may have been exposed to HIV, contact your provider immediately. Time is of the essence. Also, if you are HIV negative and in a relationship with someone who is HIV positive, discuss this directly with your provider so you can take the best possible precautions (CDC, 2016).

5. **Minimize your use of alcohol and drugs**. Alcohol and drugs can lower inhibitions and make it easier to engage in riskier sexual behavior. Moderate or eliminate your use of drugs and alcohol if you are going to be sexual with someone.

Resource Box

- Search the provider directory on the GLMA Health Professionals Advancing LGBTQ Equality website
- Search for health resources for the GBTQI Community on the website for the Centers for Disease Control and Prevention
- Explore the website for the Los Angeles LGBT Center and their Audre Lorde Health Program

Feuerborn©2020

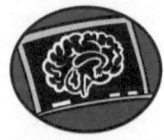 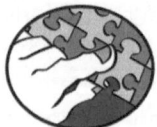

SEXUAL HEALTH CHECKLIST: GBTQI COMMUNITY

This handout was designed as a psychoeducational tool to assist in making decisions related to developing a support around one's sexual health.

Sexual health according to the World Health Organization (Savoy, O' Gurek, & Brown-James, 2020), in relation to human sexuality, is a state of physical, mental, and social well-being. Positive sexual health requires a respectful approach to sexuality and sexual relationships. Positive sexual health is free of coercion, discrimination, and violence. Conditions include the possibility of having pleasurable and safe sexual experiences.

Therapists must be comfortable in asking questions and generating a discussion around these issues in order to help clients maintain optimal health.

Following is a sexual health checklist (Winn, 2012):

1. **Discuss your sex life with your medical provider**. Your provider needs to know your sexuality and the type of sex you engage in because it will help them to order the proper tests and help you maintain optimal health. If you do not feel comfortable talking about these issues with your provider, you can role play this with a therapist before talking to your doctor; or find a provider with whom you feel more comfortable (Winn, 2012).

2. **Know your HIV status and get proper treatment**. This is important for everyone, especially if you have been or are currently sexually active. The human immunodeficiency virus (HIV) is the virus that causes AIDS. Men who have sex with men are at a higher risk for contracting HIV. HIV is transmitted through anal or vaginal sex without a condom or without medications to prevent or treat HIV. For someone who is HIV-negative, anal-receptive sex (bottoming) is the riskiest behavior. Topping (anal-insertive sex) can also pose a risk.

   Tremendous advances have been made in recent years which make HIV a more chronic and manageable disease, not a death sentence. But you must know your status and get treatment, or it remains very dangerous. If you are HIV positive, you should receive medical treatment from an HIV specialist, rather than simply a general practitioner or family doctor (Toren, 2018).

3. **Protect yourself from HIV/AIDS**. Several medications are used now to prevent HIV infection for those at risk. Pre-exposure prophylaxis (PrEP) is typically one pill, once-per-day, that can significantly reduce the likelihood of contracting HIV if you have sex with someone who is HIV positive. Additionally, post-exposure prophylaxis (PEP) is a similar protocol that can prevent infection after potential exposure. Talk to your doctor about PrEP or PEP. If your doctor is not willing to prescribe the medications, talk to another provider. Most insurance companies, including public insurance, will pay for PrEP and PEP. The pharmaceutical companies have a co-payment assistance program, so typically the medication will not cost you anything. Many county funded health providers and clinics also provide free intervention. If you believe you may have been exposed to HIV, contact your provider immediately. Time is of the essence. Also, if you are HIV negative and in a relationship with someone who is HIV positive, discuss this directly with your provider so you can take the best possible precautions (CDC, 2016; Winn, 2012).

4. **Talk with sex partners about STIs and getting tested**. Make sure you talk about sexually transmitted infections and testing – before you have sex with someone (CDC, 2016).

5. **Understand safer sex and practice it**. Condoms are an important tool to protect you from sexually transmitted infections, including HIV/AIDS, human papilloma virus (HPV), hepatitis, herpes, gonorrhea, chlamydia, and syphilis. Protect yourself by using condoms, especially when you do not know much about your sexual partner's history (CDC, 2016; Winn, 2012).

6. **Get the right tests**. The Centers for Disease Control (2016) recommends gay men, bisexual men, and other men who have sex with men to be tested at least yearly for HIV, syphilis, and hepatitis B and C. Also, regular testing for chlamydia and gonorrhea is necessary and should include additional swab tests of the throat, anus, and genital area (CDC, 2016; Winn, 2012).

7. **Get vaccinated**. Vaccines exist for various types of hepatitis and HPV. Talk to your doctor about these vaccines. A flu or COVID-19 vaccine is an added measure of protection (CDC, 2016; Winn, 2012).

8. **Minimize your use of alcohol and drugs**. Alcohol and drugs can lower inhibitions and make it easier to engage in riskier sexual behavior. Moderate or eliminate your use of drugs and alcohol if you are going to be sexual with someone (CDC, 2016).

9. **Be aware if you are acting compulsively with sex and seek help if necessary**. Problematic Sexual Behavior (PSB) exists when a person's "consensual sexual urges, thoughts, and behaviors lead to troublesome consequences" (Kort, 2018, p. 203). Having a lot of sex or a high sex drive does not mean that PSB exists. There's nothing wrong with masturbation, pornography use, or BDSM. Instead, it's important to look at the potential consequences of the behavior. Ask yourself, "Is my sexual behavior causing me problems in my relationship? Problems at work or school? Problems with friends? Has my health been affected by my sexual behavior?"

   Sexual Compulsives Anonymous (SCA) is a 12-step group dedicated to helping the LGBTQ community cope with and recover from sexually compulsive behavior. Gay, bisexual, transmen, and queer and intersex persons should stay away from Sexaholics Anonymous (SA) as it tends to be intolerant and shaming of sexuality that is not strictly heterosexual.

10. **Get appropriate cancer screenings**. Are at risk for testicular, prostate, and colon cancer, as well as other types of cancer. Screenings can occur at different points during one's lifespan. Discuss these screenings with your medical provider. Gay, bisexual, intersex persons, trans individuals, and queer men, as well as men who have sex with men, may be at greater risk for certain types of cancer. HPV, which causes anal and genital warts, can lead to anal cancer in men (Winn, 2012).

Resource Box

- Search the provider directory on the GLMA Health Professionals Advancing LGBTQ Equality website
- Search for health resources for the GBTQI Community on the website for the Centers for Disease Control and Prevention
- Explore the topic of sexual health and HIV/AIDS on the World Health Organization website
- Check-out the web resources for Pets Are Wonderful Support Los Angeles (PAWS/LA), AIDS Healthcare Foundation, and AIDS Project Los Angeles

Feuerborn©2020

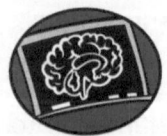 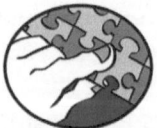

SEXUAL HEALTH CHECKLIST: TRANS COMMUNITY

This handout was designed as a psychoeducational tool to assist in making decisions related to developing a support around one's sexual health.

Sexual health according to the World Health Organization (Savoy, O' Gurek, & Brown-James, 2020), in relation to human sexuality, is a state of physical, mental, and social well-being. Positive sexual health requires a respectful approach to sexuality and sexual relationships. Positive sexual health is free of coercion, discrimination, and violence. Conditions include the possibility of having pleasurable and safe sexual experiences.

Therapists must be comfortable in asking questions and generating a discussion around these issues in order to help clients maintain optimal health.

Following is a sexual health checklist (Allison, 2012):

1. **Find a medical provider with whom you are comfortable**. Many trans people delay or avoid preventative health care, such as pelvic or colon exams or testing for sexually transmitted infections, due to fear of discrimination or disrespect. If you are uncomfortable with your provider, find another provider. Consider going to a clinic that specializes in helping trans persons (Allison, 2012).

2. **Tell your provider about your health and medical history**. Tell your provider about medications and surgeries. Also discuss your sexual history including whom you are sexual with. The more your physician or provider knows about you, the better health care they can provide (Allison, 2012).

3. **Discuss hormone treatment (if appropriate for you)**. Only take hormones that are being provided and monitored by your physician or medical provider. Trans women should discuss estrogen and understand health risks to be aware of. Trans men should discuss testosterone and associated risks. Tests for appropriate hormone levels are necessary to ensure you are not taking too much or too little (Allison, 2012).

4. **Get screened for cancer**. While hormone treatment does not usually cause cancer, it is important to discuss risks with your doctor. You also should be regularly screened for reproductive cancers; so discuss this with your provider as well (Allison, 2012).

5. **Practice safer sex and get the right tests**. Sexually active trans individuals are at risk for sexually transmitted infections, including HIV (human immunodeficiency virus, the virus that causes AIDS), HPV (human papilloma virus), hepatitis, gonorrhea, chlamydia, and syphilis. Talk to your provider about your risk factors for STIs (Allison, 2012; CDC, 2016).

6. **Protect yourself from HIV/AIDS**. Several medications are used now to prevent HIV infection for those at risk. Pre-exposure prophylaxis (PrEP) is typically one pill, once-per-day, that can significantly reduce the likelihood of contracting HIV if you have sex with someone who is HIV positive. Additionally, post-exposure prophylaxis (PEP) is a similar protocol that can prevent infection after potential exposure. Talk to your doctor about PrEP or PEP. If your doctor is not willing to prescribe the medications, talk to another provider. Most insurance companies, including public insurance, will pay for PrEP and PEP. The pharmaceutical

companies have a co-payment assistance program, so typically the medication will not cost you anything. Many county funded health providers and clinics also provide free intervention. If you believe you may have been exposed to HIV, contact your provider immediately. Time is of the essence. Also, if you are HIV negative and in a relationship with someone who is HIV positive, discuss this directly with your provider so you can take the best possible precautions (CDC, 2016).

7. **Talk with sex partners about STIs and getting tested**. Make sure you talk about sexually transmitted infections and testing – before you have sex with someone (CDC, 2016).

8. **Understand safer sex and practice it**. Condoms are an important tool to protect you from sexually transmitted infections, including HIV/AIDS, human papilloma virus (HPV), hepatitis, herpes, gonorrhea, chlamydia, and syphilis. Protect yourself by using condoms, especially when you do not know much about your sexual partner's history (CDC, 2016).

9. **Minimize your use of alcohol and drugs**. Alcohol and drugs can lower inhibitions and make it easier to engage in riskier sexual behavior. Moderate or eliminate your use of drugs and alcohol if you are going to be sexual with someone (Allison, 2012).

Resource Box

- Check-in with the website for the National Center for Transgender Equality
- Search the trans health provider directory on the GLMA Health Professionals Advancing LGBTQ Equality website
- Explore the websites and resources offered by the CARE Center in Long Beach, San Francisco AIDS Foundation, and the Center of Excellence for Transgender Health at the University of California at San Francisco

Feuerborn©2020

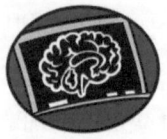

YOUR LGBTQI BRAIN

LGBTQI community members are more likely to experience potentially traumatizing events, mental and physical health problems, and discrimination throughout their lifetime compared to heterosexuals according to the research. Studies on the impact of traumatic events on the mental health and functioning of LGBTQI individuals highlight the importance of providing a safe, sexually affirming space in mental health treatment for LGBTQI individuals. This research is additionally important especially if clients are receiving treatment related to traumatic events. Individuals must ensure they are comfortable coming out to their therapists. Therapist must be skilled at addressing negative ideas related to LGBTQI identity in session and teaching effective coping skills for stressors related to discrimination. These strategies have been found to be effective for improving treatment outcomes for members of the LGBTQI community (Scheer, Harney, Esposito, & Woulfe, 2019).

We must be mindful of how LGBTQI experiences of traumatic events (e.g., the alarming murder of trans people in the world with Brazil ranking the most frightening), including historical trauma, impacts neurobiology, and the three parts of our brains in different ways than it does our heterosexual counterparts. Often, LGBTQI trauma keeps us in our reptile brain or cerebellum, where one feels the intensity of the *flight* or *fight* response. The impact of minority stress must also be evaluated.

Check out *The Three Main Parts of Your Brain* by Dr. Russ Harris on YouTube.

Directions: As you self-reflect on your life experiences, which of the three brain regions was activated during the particular memory you may recall? Were you in *flight* mode and in your Reptile Brain, were you experiencing nostalgia and thinking about a fun memory and in your Limbic System Brain, or were you in your Neocortex Brain and using abstract thought to reason and problem-solve? Using the infographic, write down in the space provided examples of thinking patterns or behaviors that were reflective of the part of the brain you were in at that time.

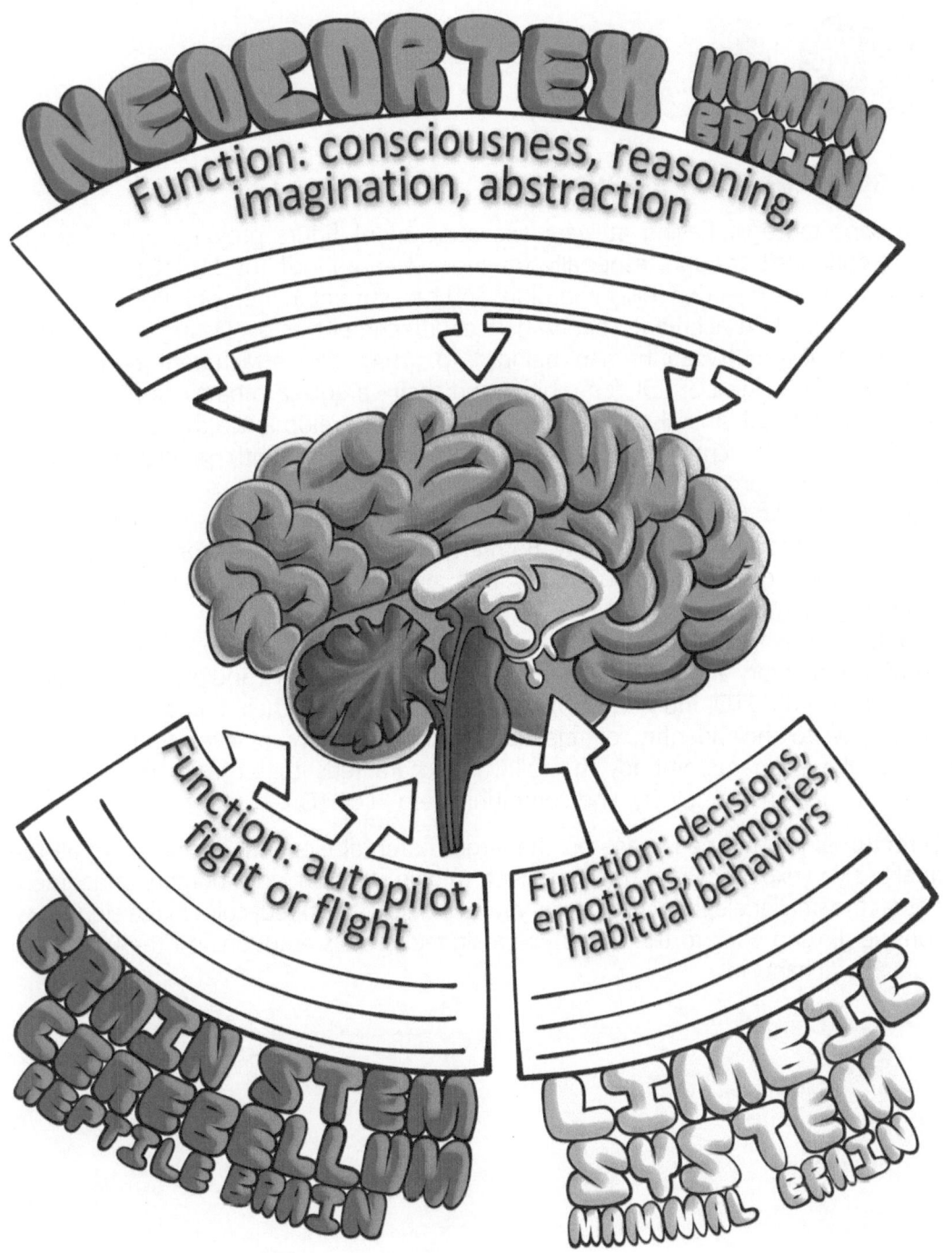

NEOCORTEX HUMAN BRAIN

Function: consciousness, reasoning, imagination, abstraction

Function: autopilot, fight or flight

Function: decisions, emotions, memories, habitual behaviors

BRAIN STEM CEREBELLUM REPTILE BRAIN

LIMBIC SYSTEM MAMMAL BRAIN

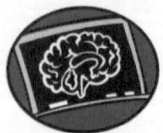 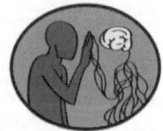

ATTACHMENT BOND ELEPHANTS

The importance of having at least one attachment figure growing up cannot be overemphasized enough, especially for those members of the LGBTQI community who often face rejection, discrimination, and harassment in life. John Bowlby (1969), the founder of Attachment Theory, defines attachment as a "lasting psychological connectedness between human beings" (p. 194). The attachment between an individual from the LGBTQI community and their caregiver impacts all relationships beyond childhood, and also impacts one's ability to develop a healthy self-esteem.

Check out Dr. Schott's podcast on *Attachment Theory* with Sir Richard Bowlby (John Bowlby's son) and Dr. Pat Sable on YouTube.

Elephants, like humans, live long lives. We both cherish relationships and families. They grieve loss in their community. Both elephant and human offspring have longer than average developmental periods that nurture and build skills essential for independent living.

Both species live in communities and can have families or tribes. We both have emotional memory and feel similar emotions; they can feel love and protective feelings like humans. LGBTQI individuals may face rejection from their primary attachment figure due to their identity, or rejection from community, or even worse. Human beings like elephants embody the following characteristics: Concern over parental care, companionship, loyalty, and community (e.g., LGBTQI).

Directions: In the open space on the larger parental elephant, write down all the qualities you experienced or feel you need to gain still from your primary attachment figure (the smaller elephant represents you as a child). If inspired, color in the elephants; consider linking back to the colors you assigned various emotions on the Emotional Color Coral handout.

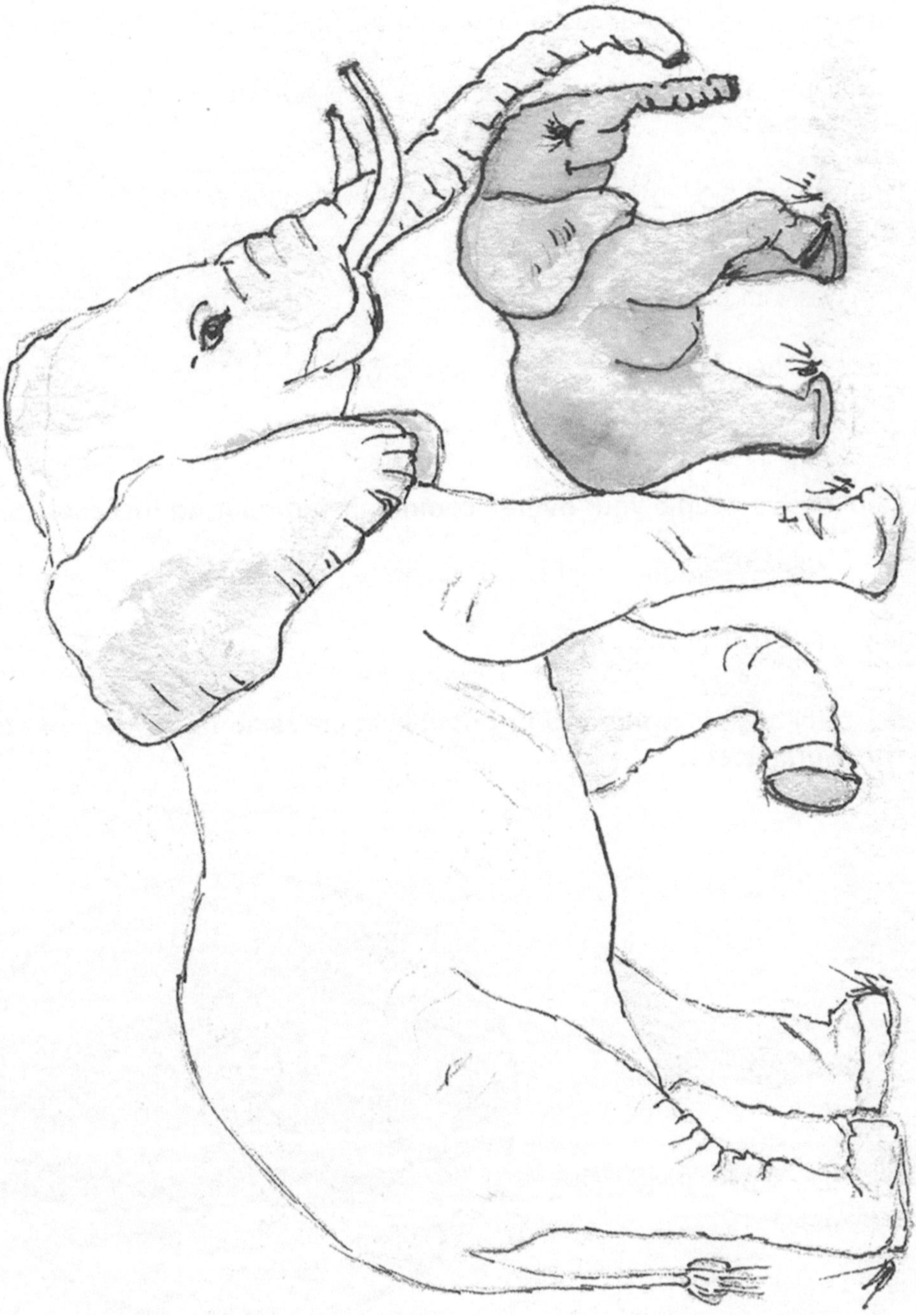

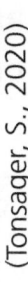
(Tonsager, S., 2020)

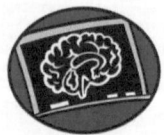 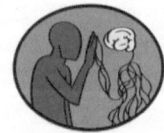

RELATIONSHIP VALIDATION CHECKLIST

Directions: Couple is to self-reflect and execute the following together once a day:

- Identify the physical, non-verbal, and/or verbal validation you gave to your partner today:

- Identify the physical, non-verbal, and/or verbal validation you received from your partner today:

- What was your emotional response (how it felt to give or receive validation?):

- Reflect on theme(s) of conversation (do this with your partner, then write down response):

Self-evaluate as a couple your overall communication during this exercise:

Poor   Fair   Good   Excellent

Why did you as a couple select this rating?

Please identify any strengths and/or possible improvements for the next time using this worksheet:

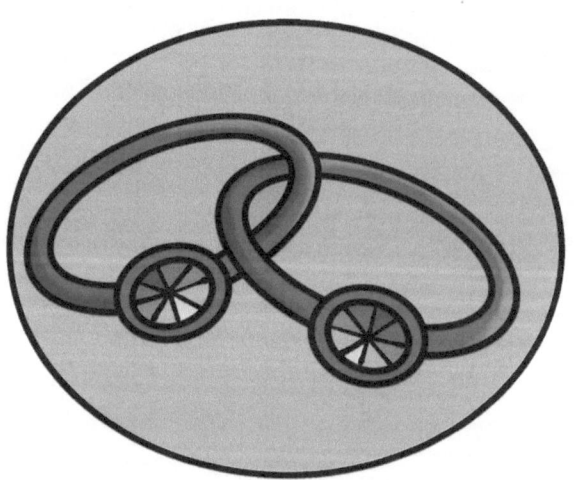

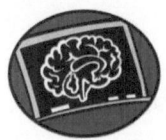

FINDING AN LGBTQI AFFIRMING THERAPIST

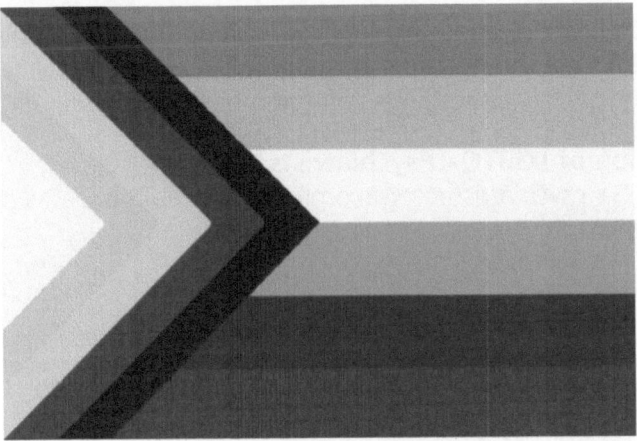

LGB individuals are three times as more likely than heterosexuals to experience a mental health condition. LGBTQ people are at a higher risk for suicidal thoughts and suicide attempts (compared to heterosexuals). According to the National Alliance on Mental Illness, 48% of all transgender adults report that they have considered suicide (compared to 4% of the overall US population). We must do better at getting sexual minorities the affirming therapies the community requires. Talking to an LGBTQI identified therapist may be a great way to establish a sense of safety. Accessing therapy outside of insurance can be expensive. Finding the right therapy can be a daunting task. There may be free or sliding scale services available at your county health department or local non-profit mental health agency or clinic, or telehealth could be an option in more rural or crisis settings, or for convenience or accessibility.

If you're in immediate danger such as harming yourself or someone else, don't wait to find a therapist – immediately call 911 or go the local emergency room.

Resources for LGBTQI Affirming Crisis Hotlines

National Suicide Prevention Lifeline
(800) 273-8255

The Trevor Project (for LGBTQ+ youth ages 13–24)
(866) 488-7386

The Gay, Lesbian, Bisexual and Transgender National Hotline
(888) 843-4564

Trans Lifeline
(877) 565-8860

National Resources

Psychology Today
Most in-depth directory with filters to narrow search by the therapist's LGBTQI specialty, modality, insurance/payment, and zip code

The National Queer and Trans Therapist of Color Network
Resources and directory of therapists across the USA

GLMA: Health Professionals Advancing LGBTQ Equality (previously known as the Gay & Lesbian Medical Association)
National listings of queer and queer-affirming health professionals

The Association of LGBTQ+ Psychiatrists
National LGBTQ+ psychiatrist referral organization that educates and advocates on LGBTQ+ mental health issues

State/City Resources
Gaylesta (San Francisco)
Lighthouse (New York)
Manhattan Alternatives (New York)
The LGBT-Affirmative Therapist Guild
LAGPA (Los Angeles)
LGBTQ Therapist Resource (Georgia)
Seattle Counseling Service (Washington)

Local LGBTQI Centers
Center Link (National Directory of LGBTQ Community Centers)
LA LGBT Center (Los Angeles, California)
Center on Halstead (Chicago, Illinois)
The Center on Colfax (Denver, Colorado)
Pridelines Miami's LGBTQ Community Center (Florida)
The Center (New York)
The LGBTQ Center of Southern Nevada (Las Vegas, Nevada)
The LGBT Center of St. Louis (Missouri)
CAMP Rehoboth Community Center (Rehoboth Beach, Delaware)
Hudson Valley LGBTQ Center (Kingston, New York)

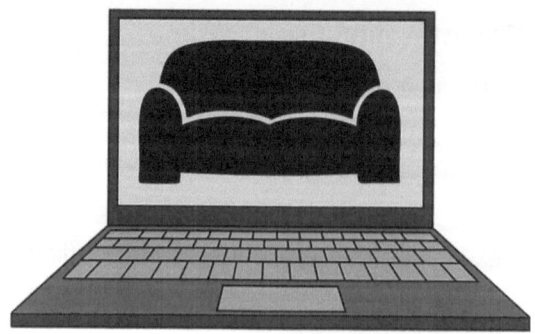

Telehealth
Talkspace
Pride Counseling
Better Help
USC Telehealth Online Clinic

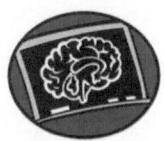

PREPARING FOR THERAPY TIPS

We all need help sometimes and getting ready for your first therapy session or returning back to therapy may be intimidating. Completing the handouts and worksheets in this workbook is a great primer for getting ready for therapy with a professional (unless you require immediate care). The following are some useful tips (with much of that data needed being obtainable within this workbook's handout and worksheets):

1. Understand the financial obligation, insurance benefits, and/or the client qualifications for the benefit source being considered. Confirm the format of service delivery (face-to-face or virtual).
2. Check the therapist's qualifications and licensure standing. Psychology Today verifies each of the licenses of the therapists in their directory. You can also check your state's licensing boards. For example, in California, do a DCA license search to check to see if a potential therapist has a license in good standing. The State of California Board of Behavioral Sciences offers a resource on empowerment in the process of finding a mental health professional.
3. Gather all relevant documents such as medical and psychiatric records, hospital discharge summaries, educational testing, or the Biological-Psychological-Social AT Assessment form in the Appendix of this workbook. Complete the agency's, clinic's, or provider's intake paperwork prior to your first session if possible.
4. Have all the details of your medications documented (if applicable). This includes the details of the name of medication, dose, and purpose. Include prescription medication, as well as anything over the counter you may be taking, and/or alternative medication, homeopathy, or herbal treatments.
5. Take detailed notes leading up to your first session to help remind you of the questions you hope to have clarified.
6. Plan your calendar for the frequency and duration of the treatment you have planned with your therapist. Make sure you are setting realistic and achievable goals.

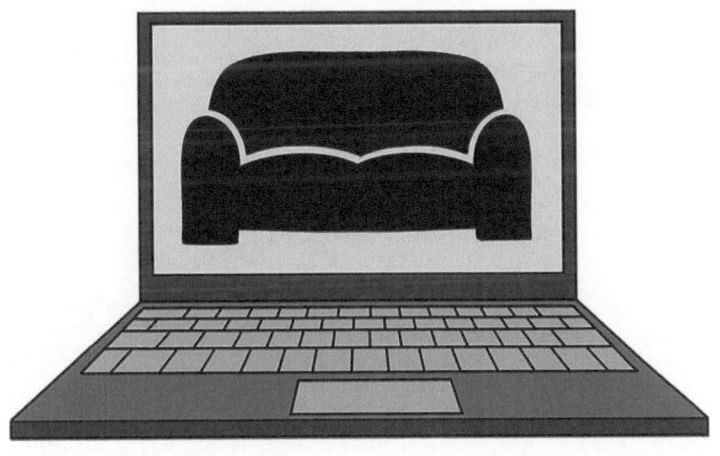

Part 5

Therapist Handouts and Worksheets

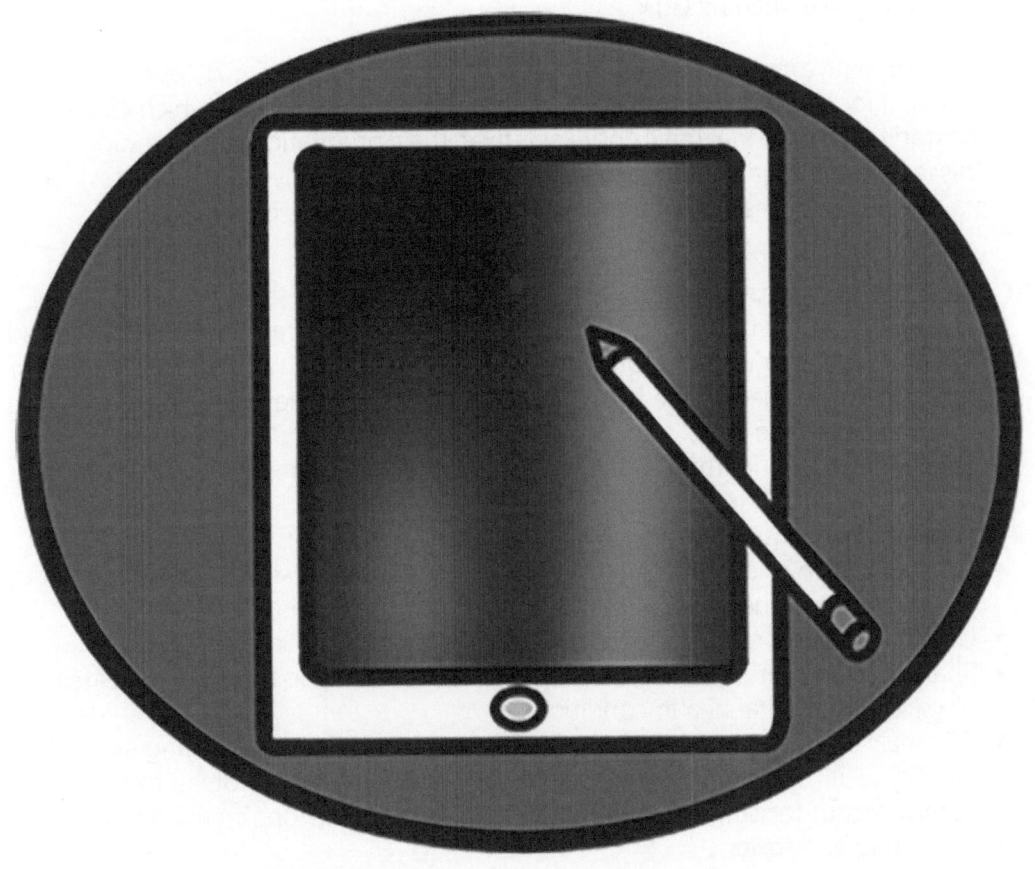

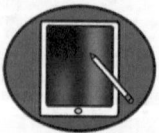

LGBTQI AFFIRMATIVE THERAPY (AT)

The first definition of Gay Affirmative Psychotherapy (Maylon, 1982), now called LGBTQI Affirmative Therapy (AT):

> Gay affirmative psychotherapy is not an independent system of psychotherapy. Rather, it represents a special range of psychological knowledge which challenges the traditional view that [gay] desire and fixed [gay] orientations are pathological…. This approach regards homophobia, as opposed to [gayness/queerness], as a major variable in the development of certain symptomatic conditions.
>
> (pp. 68–69)

AT Therapist Competency Checklist:
- LGBTQI identified therapists and straight therapists alike can both be uninformed when it comes to the LGBTQI community – pledge right now to always try your best to be informed of the issues of the day and how they were informed from experiences of the past;
- Sexual identity (orientation) is who we love and to whom we are attracted to or not;
- Gender identity is about who we believe ourselves to be;
- An AT clinician understands and respects the identity of sex and assigned sex at birth (reference The LGBTQI Identity Iguana infographic handout);
- Understands and respects the identity of genderqueer/non-binary/GNC clients;
- Shame-based cultures are not good for self-esteem or the risk it creates for physical and mental health conditions;
- AT's main stance is that there is nothing inherently wrong with having an LGBTQI identity – it is not the individual but rather the homophobia, transphobia, heterosexism, racism, misogynism, and xenophobia in one's environment that are wrong and toxic;
- AT's goal is to repair these environmental wrongs and build on the client's strengths from a resiliency framework;
- Getting the client or group to experience moments of one's authentic sense-of-self that is prideful rather than shame-based;
- AT is a framework, like Ecological Systems Theory (Brofenbrenner, 1989), that informs psychotherapy, it is not an intervention;
- The job of an AT therapist sometimes is to educate the client of their LGBTQI history and current issues (reference LGBTQI History handout, LGBTQI Terminology handout);
- Creating (in collaboration with the client) an environment that provides healthy corrective emotional experiences is essential in treatment with clients that identify as LGBTQI;
- Validation is a critical therapeutic skill for any competent therapist, if you make a mistake, apologize and continue with treatment, staying client-centered;
- Creating a life worth living for while at the same time acknowledging the personal and/or historical traumas of the past is key in this framework;
- A competent AT therapist will understand heterosexism and actively work to fight against its existence when uncovered or spotted;

- Understanding heterosexual and cisgender privilege is essential and how it impacts institutional freedoms, legal rights and protections, and societal freedoms;
- For some clients there could be a bereavement of losing heterosexual or cisgender privilege;
- Clients may have also experienced additional personal loss (family, work, friends, etc.) due to coming out;
- Be mindful of misdiagnosis or overdiagnosis (complicated grief, major depressive disorder [MDD], adjustment disorder, generalized anxiety disorder [GAD], borderline personality disorder [BPD], post-traumatic stress disorder [PTSD], acute stress disorder, body dysmorphic disorder, bulimia nervosa, anorexia nervosa);
- Borderline Personality Disorder (BPD) may have been over-diagnosed historically in the LGBTQI community (Eubanks-Carter & Goldfried, 2006);
- Do not alienate, validate!

Self-Reflection:

Using the Identity Iguana infographic, how might you describe your individual identity regarding:

Sex or Assigned Sex at Birth:

Sexual Identity (Orientation):

Gender Identity:

Gender Expression:

Next, Consider the Following:

List three steps you have taken or can take to make spaces more LGBTQI inclusive:

List three validations you will give out during your sessions with clients:

Using the Emotional Color Coral handout, how do you imagine you might feel after giving these three validations?

And for your client?

Finally, doing a body scan where do you notice the afore feeling or emotion resonating in your body right now (reference the Grounding Technique: Body Scan handout and worksheet)?

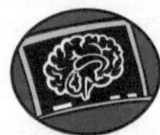

INTERSEX AFFIRMATIVE THERAPY (IAT)

Bereavement, trauma, identity development, social and familial support, loneliness, isolation, shame, and guilty are themes of concerns that often bring intersex clients into therapy (Alderson, 2013).

IAT Therapist Competency Checklist:

- Limited research on counseling strategies for intersex individuals, typically qualitative (case studies) and theoretical.
- In 2020, the first national study of intersex adults in the USA was conducted using community-based research methods to describe the health of intersex adults (Rosenwohl-Mack, et al., 2020). Alarmingly, over 43% of participants in this research rated one's physical health as fair or poor and 53% reported fair or poor mental health. Over half of the 198 participants reported serious difficulties with cognitive tasks and nearly a third reported difficulty with everyday life tasks (Rosenwohl-Mack, et al., 2020).
- Prevalent health diagnoses for intersex people included depression, anxiety, arthritis, and hypertension, with significant differences by age (Rosenwohl-Mack, et al., 2020).
- It is essential, to gain a greater understanding of intersex health over the life spectrum. More longitudinal studies and further examination of potential health disparities experienced by intersex people are needed to inform better intersex affirmative and competent care.
- Counseling strategies could include the following:
  - Empathic, sensitive, and attuned support;
  - Psychoeducation to facilitate an understanding of intersex for individuals regarding physical development and/or psychosocial identity development (Sanders, Carter, & Lwin, 2015);
  - Counselors should always explore identity development as individual and evolving and never forget where a client is in the different spheres of their lives;
  - Psychoeducation to facilitate understanding for families;
  - Resources must be specialized and tailored to your client's or community's needs; one's local resource or LGBTQ community center may not be a place their client feels welcome;
  - Counselors should always take a strengths-based or empowerment framework when working with families to assist them in making the best possible choices regarding a minor's medical care; advocacy within medical and mental health systems of care may also be a key role the counselor takes on;
  - Counselors should always dynamically assess for the following when working with their clients:
    - Ethnic and racial identity;
    - Minority stress impact;
    - Education and family history;

- Schemas about sexuality, both within the family at the micro-level of assessment, the community at the mezzo, and then the macro cultural view of sexuality;
- Secrets and family silence may also need to be the focus of clinical attention;
- Common in the LGBTQI community is the issue of shame; internalized and externalized feelings must be addressed by the counselor (reference Checking Toxic Shame handout); other common feelings that may need to be processed in treatment could be anger and betrayal;
- Attachment bonds and the impact on family systems remaining balanced or trauma-inflicted is a crucial assessment piece; an ACE score assessment is optimal (reference Attachment Bonds handout and worksheet).

An affirmative, relational-cultural, abolitionist, feminist, and queer integrated approach is the recommended stance for a competent AT to take and could include the following (Richmond, Burnes, Singh, & Ferrara, 2017):

- Provide psychoeducation;
- Acknowledge clients' feelings, validate oppression, do not over-pathologize;
- View may be that the medical community as a whole is untrustworthy and victimizes people;
- Build rapport;
- Promote transparency in assessment and diagnosis, address expectations both medically and in psychotherapy;
- Improve communication, if needed address surgery and identity discussion;
- Develop trust in the professional counseling relationship, which will be fundamental to any strategy;
- Allow individuals to voice their feelings, concerns, and reactions;
- Provide a reading list and media and/or video resources if appropriate;
- Have the intersex pride sticker on your door or phone/computer;
- Celebrate and acknowledge that October 26 is Intersex Awareness Day (Herculine Barbin's birthday);
- Understand who Herculine Barbin (1838–1868) was;
- Intersex affirming therapists should learn that using the identity label of *sex* is more inclusive to many intersex people as one's *assigned sex at birth* (ASAB) was often not intersex for most in their personal experiences. An intersex person's true sex is *intersex* but are often assigned male or female at birth (AMAB or AFAB). Assigned sex at birth is a source of trauma and struggle for many as surgeries and hormones followed to affirm that assignment.

10 Collaborative Treatment Planning Suggestions:

1. Develop a positive identity;
2. Build on strengths and resiliency;
3. Help increase positive and adaptive coping skills and behaviors;
4. Work actively to counter cognitive distortions and messages of shame and guilt;
5. Use a trauma-informed care approach to treatment;
6. Where there is complex trauma, discuss the impact for clients, and refer for evidence-based practices like EMDR, Cognitive Processing Therapy (CPT), or Seeking Safety, with the main goal being hopefully a reduction in mental health symptoms;

7. Teach communication and self-advocacy skills with the goal being empowerment;
8. Provide resources of websites of intersex advocacy groups;
9. Reduce feelings of isolation;
10. Identify and link to support groups, psychotherapy groups, and online resources (Ginicola, Smith, & Filmore, 2017).

Resource Box

- Find the complete toolkit for intersex education and awareness on the website #4Intersex
- Checkout the American Library Association (ALA) website on professional tools and intersex resources
- Discover readings and resources on the interACT website
- Explore the InterConnect and cxycourtney.com websites for resources and advocacy information

---

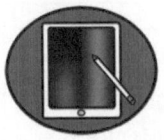 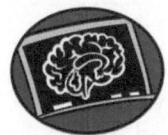

TRANS AFFIRMATIVE THERAPY (TAT)

Trans is a broad term. It can be used to describe people whose gender identity is different from the gender they were thought to be when given at birth. Respectful treatment of trans individuals means that one treats them according to their gender identity, not their sex or assigned sex at birth. Trans people have always been part of the LGBTQI civil rights movement, with such pioneers as Marsha P. Johnson. Explore the interactive website from the New York Times called Overlooked which highlights a series of obituaries about remarkable people, like Marsha, whose deaths, beginning in 1851, went unreported in the paper.

Ally etiquette:

- Always call a person by their proper name and pronoun;
- Just ask someone how they would like to be addressed if you are not sure;
- When asking about pronouns, avoid the use of the word "preferred" as it implies somehow that there is a choice or another option for a gender identity;
- Apologize quickly if you mispronoun or get a name wrong and move on, do not make the other individual have to console you on your mistake;
- Interrogative questioning is not a trauma-informed approach to effective communication and is not a recommended approach for therapists to take with their trans clients;
- Most trans clients do not necessarily want to discuss their gender identity constantly;
- Asking a person if they identify as pre-op or post-op is offensive language and should never be asked;
- Just merely asking if someone is trans can be seen as an aggressive behavior depending on context;
- These are offensive and abusive terms: transgendered, tranny, he-she, she-male, transvestite, hermaphrodite, sex change, sexual reassignment surgery, passing, stealth;
- Not all trans people identify as being part of the LGBTQI community;
- The trans community should not be sexualized;
- Never ask a trans or intersex person if they have had surgery;
- Questions about bodies is OK, but only if it links to the reasons for seeking treatment from a therapist or provider;
- Pronoun inclusion in email signatures can help promote inclusivity and increase visibility;
- Asking pronouns in group settings (e.g., club, work, school) may force individuals to disclose when there could be risks to personal safety or activation of past trauma;
- Other identities could include genderqueer, non-binary, GNC, gender-fluid, or bi-gender;
- Trans identity is about one's gender identity, not sexual orientation or attraction – remember, we all have a gender and sexual identity, male heterosexuality tends to be the dominant narrative researched historically;
- Sexual identity (orientation) for trans persons possibly could include queer, straight, gay, lesbian, asexual, or pansexual;
- Ask for example: "What is your pronoun? What is your name? Regarding your gender identity, how would you like to be referred to?"

Resource Box

- Visit the National Center for Transgender Equality and check out their resources on supporting trans people in one's life and tips on how to be a good ally to the community
- The World Professional Association for Transgender Health (WPATH) website has legal, policy, and reading resources
- The Center of Excellence for Transgender Health website at the University of California at San Francisco has education resources
- Listen to the podcast with Brené Brown and Lavern Cox on trans representation
- Explore the American Psychological Association website for LGBTQI resources
- The Center for Transyouth Health and Development at Children's Hospital Los Angeles provides resources and information on their website

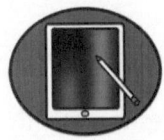

AT THERAPIST TIPS

Common missteps:

According to Kort (2018), the ten common fundamental errors a therapist makes when **not** utilizing the AT framework include:

1. Not disclosing your own sexual identity (orientation) when asked by the client or group;
2. Denying one's homophobia, transphobia, and heterosexual and cisgender privilege;
3. Not offering resources or appropriate referrals for clients;
4. Using the wrong terminology, proper name, or pronoun;
5. Using intake forms and paperwork that are heterosexist, heteronormative, racist, transphobic, misogynistic, or xenophobic;
6. Being a blank slate or *tabula rasa* as a therapist never works effectively;
7. Neglecting an LGBTQI identity from a client's childhood in session is a damaging microaggression, and it could harm them – instead one could use soft and inclusive language;
8. Have a waiting room, organization group room, restroom, etc. that is completely lacking in any LGBTQI materials;
9. Making statements about being non-judgmental in treatment like: "I just love that gay marriage is here, I voted for it you know";
10. Mis-assessing where a client is on the spectrum of their identity development and in the coming out process and/or failing on the part of the therapist to ask about the social domains that may have distinct and siloed experiences (e.g., being out in one's immediate family but not being out at work).

Tips:

1. Self-reflection is essential at least once per week, consider an ongoing version of the activity from the front and back covers of this workbook by breaking it out weekly or monthly;
2. Get involved and attend an LGBTQI cultural event;
3. Create physically affirming environments, like making a pride sticker visible in your office;
4. Solidly committed to ethical service delivery to your LGBTQI clients;
5. Challenge the gender binary, homophobia, transphobia, and heterosexism when uncovered or witnessed;
6. Competent therapists always consult and challenge their countertransference issues;
7. Challenge oppression of sexual and gender minorities;
8. Obtain knowledge regarding accessing resources for the LGBTQI community;
9. Every human is a unique diamond with multiple facets that make them who they are, acknowledge this, and validate a person's journey of self-discovery;
10. Understand the identities of sex or assigned sex at birth, sexual identity (orientation), gender identity, and gender expression and be able to discuss the concepts and understand the differences using the Identity Iguana infographic;

11. Use correct terminology;
12. Intake forms and material should always have room for inclusive or blank options when asking about all identity categories;
13. Continuing education is an ethical practice for professional mental health providers, such as social workers, psychiatrist, psychologist, nurses, and licensed counselors and psychotherapists – a competent LGBTQI Affirming Therapist accesses LGBTQI Affirmative Therapy training, supervision, and reads books and workbooks regularly;
14. Work to actively abolish Conversion Therapy and protect clients from harm always.

TRAUMA-INFORMED CARE (TIC) CHECKLIST

Trauma is extensive in the LGBTQI community – up to 95% of women in public health systems of care report some history of trauma. Addressing trauma in your psychotherapy practice, clinic, or agency improves the quality and impact of mental health services for the LGBTQI community who have experience historical traumas. Taking a trauma-informed care approach to treatment increases safety, reduces missed appointments, enhances client engagement and rapport with the therapist, and avoids burnout and turnover. When a provider misses the opportunity to inquire about a client's trauma history and current experiences, they may create harm or abuse unintentionally and retraumatize them by the use of forced medications, restraints, or isolation (Scheer, Harney, Esposito, & Woulfe, 2019).

According to the Maryland Network Against Domestic Violence website, a trauma-informed clinician and organization must adhere to the following checklist based on the 12 Elements of Trauma-Informed Care (McKinnish, Burgess, & Sloan, 2019):

- Maintain a non-judgmental view on the ways in which the client has attempted to cope;
- Allow the client to have control over the process – provide feedback, make decisions, even to stop;
- Remember and affirm that healing looks different for each client, and do not assume what will be easy or difficult for them in their recovery;
- Validate their clients' responses to trauma, which are legitimate regardless of the details of their story;
- Understand *fight, flight,* and *freeze* responses and how the nervous system can be rebalanced;
- Invite their client to establish a clear connection to the *here and now* with a variety of practices they can use before, during, and after treatment;
- Help strengthen their client's verbal and nonverbal communication by collaborating and engaging with them during the treatment;
- Provide ample opportunities for their client to practice making firm, clear, self-directed choices;
- Recognize and attend to how sexual violence intersects with other forms of violence and systems of oppression;
- Plan ahead for triggers and flashbacks in the practice space, and develop tools to orient, ground, and soothe their client;
- Work with and refer out to a multidisciplinary team, staying very clearly within their own scope of practice;
- Prioritize their own self-care as essential, not optional.

Resource Box

- Download the trauma and resiliency informed care toolkit from the Downtown Women's Center website
- Check out Rainbow Services in Southern California for resources and services to address intimate partner violence
- Read about the 12 elements of TIC on the Breathe Network website

---

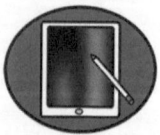

CONVERSION THERAPY BANS

Conversion Therapy (CT) is a harmful and discredited therapy practice directed at reversing or changing one's same-sex romantic, physical, or emotional attractions. It is a dangerous attempt at "curing" one from their LGBTQI identity. Therapists practicing this method use shame, torture, psychological abuse, and physically painful stimuli to try to force their patient victims to give up their LGBTQI identity. The image below shows a shock machine from the ONE Archives at the University of Southern California that was used in CT. The torture device would be connected to a patient's body, allowing painful electric impulses to be administered by the therapist when the client reacted to any photos containing LGBTQI themes.

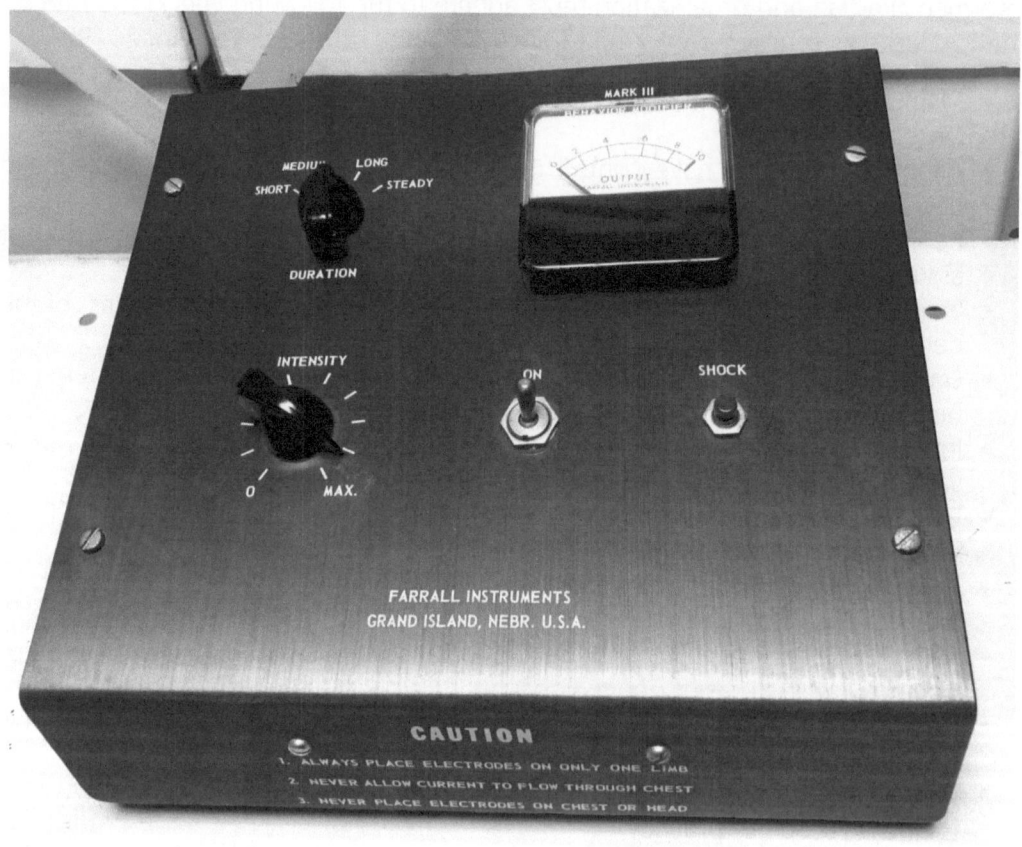

Conversion Therapy torcher machine at the ONE Archives, University of Southern California Libraries, Los Angeles, California. March 29, 2018.

As of 2021, 20 states and Washington, D.C. have laws banning CT for youth under the age of 18 years by licensed health-care professionals. Unfortunately, the laws do not cover unlicensed providers that are often religious authorities. According to prominent LGBTQ researchers Blosnich, Henderson, Coulter, Goldbach, and Meyer (2020), LGBTQ+ people who have undergone CT are almost twice as likely to attempt suicide, compared to those from the same LGBTQ+ community who had not experienced the unethical and reckless practice. Of LGBTQ+ adults, aged 18–59, seven percent have experienced CT, often at the hands of a religious authority, according to research data. Malta, Ecuador, Brazil, Taiwan, and Germany are countries with bans on CT for those under the age of 18. For additional resources, explore the Trevor Project's noble campaign *50 Bills 50 States*, which endeavors to end CT for LGBTQI youth in all 50 states.

Resource Box

- Check out the American Bar Association's Conversion Therapy Legislative Guide on their website
- Learn about the lies and dangers of CT on the Human Rights Campaign website
- Discover which states have CT bans by visiting the map from the website for the Movement Advancement Project
- Explore the Center for LGBTQ+ Health Equity on the USC Suzanne Dworak-Peck School of Social Work website for additional resources and education

---

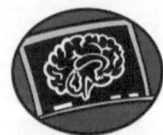 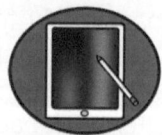

TRANS TRAUMA-INFORMED CARE

Pervasive discrimination, microaggressions, and victimization are common themes reported by members of the trans community. The impact of this trauma over the developmental lifespan contributes to disparate rates of suicide, anxiety, and depression. Trans people in the USA and around the world are being murdered at alarming rates, even more terrifying for trans persons of color. People are dying because of who they are (Dinno, 2017). Clinical interventions for trans clients should always be affirming and consider the historical traumas and triggers for the trans community. The therapist must sensitively attend to the micro effects of transphobic discrimination on the lives and experiences of trans people. Trans affirmative clinical practice acknowledges and counters the oppressive contexts from an intersectional framework (see Intersectionality Gem handout and worksheet). Historical trauma is often experienced in health and mental health care for trans clients. Experiences of trauma are frequent for trans people, often related to societal prejudice, hatred, or intolerance, because of their gender identity (Mizock & Lewis, 2008; Richmond, Burnes, & Carroll, 2012).

Five themes for the therapist to assess for and be mindful of when providing competent trauma-informed treatment for the trans community are (Burnes, Dexter, Richmond, Singh, & Cherrington, 2016):

1. Experiences of trauma within the family and/or childhood development:

2. Intrapersonal violence during transition development:

3. Interpersonal violence during transition development:

4. Experiences of trauma in public restrooms and space:

5. Protective (resiliency) and wellness (strength) factors for trans trauma survivors:

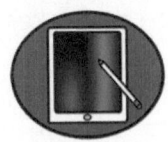 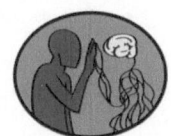

CISGENDER PRIVILEGE CHECKLIST

Cisgender is defined as having congruency between the sex you were assigned at birth and the gender you feel to be. For a person of trans identity, the opposite experience is true – there is incongruency. This checklist is a self-reflection on the privilege – the privilege that one's cisgender identity provides automatically every day for most. Members of the LGBQ and heterosexual community might consider asking themselves the 32 questions listed below to better understand one's cisgender privilege. This reflection tool is from social justice advocate Sam Killerman (2017) to help cisgender allies understand (without shame) that there are many unearned benefits that come with identifying with the gender you were assigned at birth. Allied work is about elevating other people.

Directions: Ask yourself the following 32 self-reflection questions and honestly answer if you hold this privilege, are you able to do this unquestioned. Check off how many of Killerman's (2017) cisgender privileges you hold.

- "You can use public restrooms without fear of verbal abuse, physical intimidation, or arrest.
- You can use public facilities such as gym locker rooms and store changing rooms without stares, fear, or anxiety.
- Strangers don't assume they can ask you what your genitals look like and how you have sex.
- Your validity as a man/woman/human is not based on how much surgery you've had or how well you 'pass' as non-trans.
- You can walk through the world and generally blend in, not being constantly stared or gawked at, whispered about, pointed at, or laughed at because of your gender expression.
- You can access gender-exclusive spaces (e.g., a space or activity for women), and not be excluded due to your trans status.
- Strangers call you by the name you provide and don't ask what your 'real name' (birth name) is and then assume that they have a right to call you by that name.
- You can reasonably assume that your ability to acquire a job, rent an apartment, or secure a loan will not be denied on the basis of your gender identity/ expression.
- You can flirt, engage in courtship, or form a relationship and not fear that a part of who you are may be the cause for rejection or attack, nor will it cause your partner to question their sexual orientation.
- If you end up in the emergency room, you do not have to worry that your gender will keep you from receiving appropriate treatment or that all of your medical issues will be seen as a result of your gender.
- Your identity was not formally (until 2013) considered a mental pathology ('gender identity disorder' in the DSM IV) by the psychological and medical establishments, and still pathologized by the public.
- You don't need to worry about being placed in a sex-segregated detention center, holding facility, jail, or prison that is incongruent with your identity.

- You don't have to worry about being profiled on the street as a sex worker because of your gender expression.
- You are not required to undergo an extensive psychological evaluation in order to receive basic medical care.
- You do not have to defend your right to be a part of 'queer' (or the queer community), and gays and lesbians will not try to exclude you from 'their' equal rights movement because of your gender identity (or any equality movement, including feminist rights).
- If you are murdered (or have any crime committed against you), your gender expression will not be used as a justification for your murder ('gay panic'), nor as a reason to coddle the perpetrators.
- You can easily find role models and mentors to emulate who share your identity.
- Hollywood accurately depicts people of your gender in films and television, without tokenizing your identity as the focus of a dramatic storyline or the punch line of a joke.
- You can assume that everyone you encounter will understand your identity and will not think you're confused, misled, or hell-bound when you reveal it to them.
- You can purchase clothes that match your gender identity without being refused service, mocked by staff, or questioned about your genitals.
- You can purchase shoes that fit your gender expression without having to order them in special sizes or asking someone to custom-make them.
- No stranger checking your identification or driver's license will ever insult or glare at you because your name or sex does not match the sex they believed you to be based on your gender expression.
- You can reasonably assume that you will not be denied services at a hospital, bank, or other institution because the staff does not believe the gender marker on your ID card to match your gender identity.
- Your gender is an option on a form.
- You can tick a box on a form without someone disagreeing and telling you not to lie.
- You don't have to fear interactions with police officers due to your gender identity.
- You can go places with friends on a whim knowing there will be bathrooms there you can use.
- You don't have to convince your parents of your true gender and/or have to earn your parents' and siblings' love and respect all over again because of your gender identity.
- You don't have to remind your extended family over and over to use correct gender pronouns.
- You don't have to deal with old photographs that do not reflect who you truly are.
- If you're dating someone, you know they aren't just looking to satisfy a curiosity or kink pertaining to your gender identity.
- You can pretend that anatomy and gender are irrevocably entwined when having the 'boy parts and girl parts' talk with children, instead of having to explain the actual complexity of the issue" (https://www.itspronouncedmetrosexual.com/2011/11/list-of-cisgender-privileges/, para. 3).

Score: /32

What might it feel like to not be able to do just one of these things?

How do you feel you would think if you could not do all 32?

What is one thing you can think about actioning on to become a better ally with the trans community?

Resource Box

- Review the cisgender privilege checklist on the T-Vox website
- Go over definitions related to sexual identity (orientation) and gender diversity on the American Psychological Association website

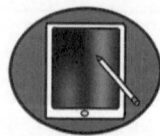 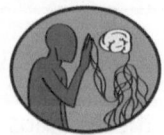

DATING SAFETY CHECKLIST

In a survey of 2,000 British singles (conducted by dating app Plenty of Fish), one in four adults said they don't know enough when it comes to dating safety, and nearly a quarter of those polled also said they were concerned for their safety while online dating (Petrecca, 2019). Not all LGBTQI individuals are out and may lack the supportive networks needed for safe dating. LGBTQ youth are at higher risk for intimate partner violence (Langenderfer-Magruder, Walls, Whitfield, Brown, & Barrett, 2016).

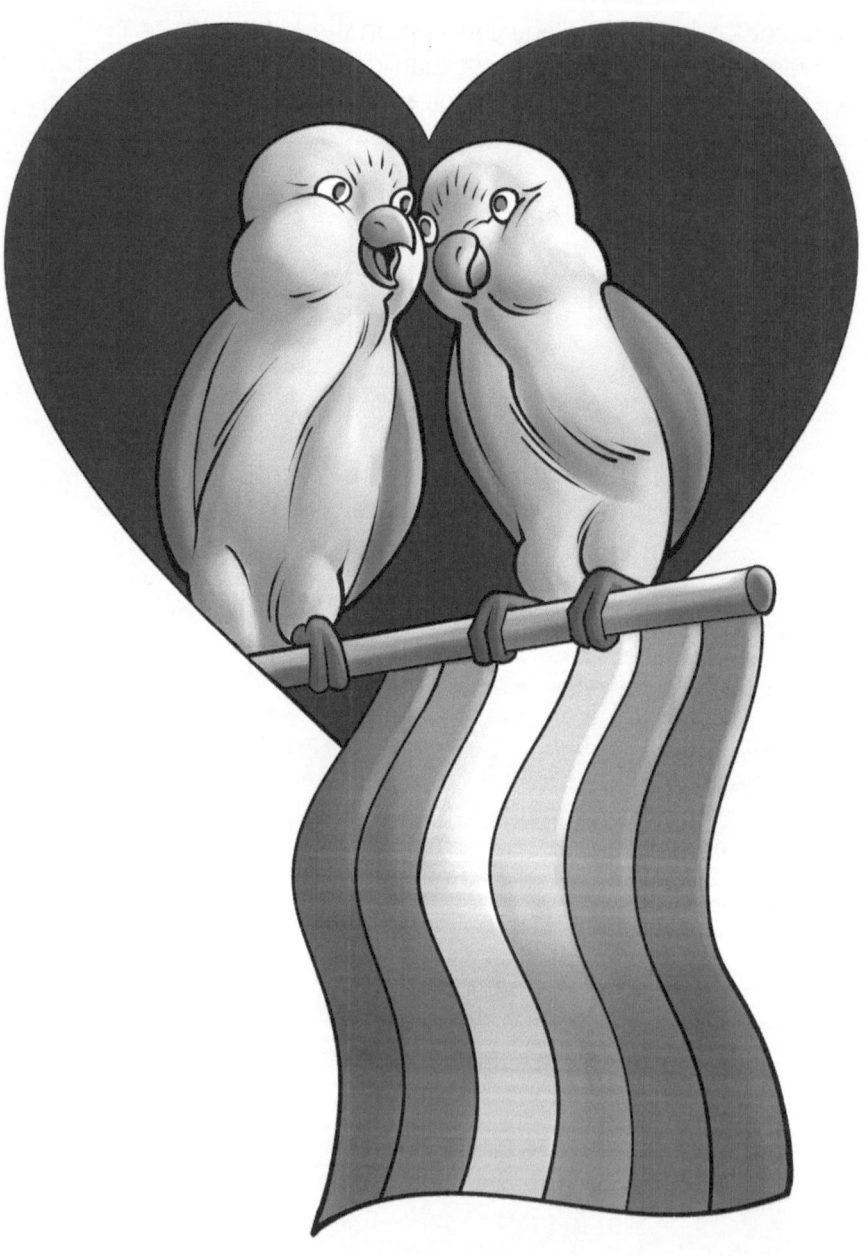

Some Tips on Dating Online from AARP:

- Play it safe and be reserved and cautious when sharing personal information.
- Always meet a potential mate first in a public setting.
- Put a premium on privacy and protect your personal data like credit cards and addresses, or social security numbers. Consider joining a premium dating site and edit out any identifying information in photos, such as a license plate number.
- Reject any requests for money as this is a red flag whenever anyone seeks cash, gift cards, merchandise, or anything else of value (if propositioned on an online dating site, report it to the dating site, and stop all communications).
- Keep conversations on the dating platform because scammers will quickly try to move the conversation to email or text, saying their subscription is about to end or they don't log onto the dating app frequently.
- Use the internet to check out your potential date by searching their social media for example.
- Investigate the images as many fraudsters cloak their real identity by using photos swiped from other sites. To discover where else a picture may have appeared, upload it to a web-scouring site that uses image recognition technology. Go to the TinEye website or do a reverse image lookup on Google.
- Set up a predate video chat as this can give you a feel for the person you are meeting – and can be done from the safety of your home (be sure to remove any personal or identifying information that could show up in the background).
- Pick a public setting for the first date like a popular hike, park, or coffee house.
- Make sure your cell phone battery is fully charged, and always provide your own transportation to and from the date; don't get into someone else's car.
- Inform friends or family of your whereabouts. Consider having a double-date or appropriate group date event – remember this may require sensitive assessment for the LGBTQI community (Petrecca, 2019).

Go to the AARP website and search for more advice from fraud experts, relationship counselors, dating sites, and consumer protection agencies.

Resource Box

- On the Hazelden Betty Ford website check out their safe dates adolescent dating abuse prevention curriculum
- Review safety tips from the University of Southern California on their USC Safety website
- Visit the CDC's website on Preventing Teen Dating Violence

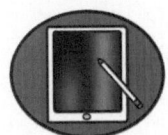

AT Progress Note

Date:

Client Information:

Session Treatment Goals:

Consideration of LGBTQI Developmental and/or Historical Trauma:

LGBTQI Affirming Sessions Themes and Positive Reinforcements:

Diagnosis: **No change** ☐

Presentation: **Stable** ☐

Cognitive functioning: **Not Assessed** ☐

Affect:

Mood:

Interpersonal:

Functional Status:

Safety Issues: **None** ☐

Suicidal Ideation and Intent, Plan, Means:

Homicidal Ideation and Intent, Plan, Means:

Medications: **No change** ☐
                                                                None ☐

Symptom Description and Subjective Report:

Relevant CBT/ABC Observations:

Cognitions (Activating Thoughts and Beliefs):

Behaviors (Consequences):

Emotions (Consequences):

Physical Sensations (Consequences):

Interventions:

Overall Observations, Goals and Objectives Review, Resources, Frequency of Visits:

Consultation, Client Conference, Interprofessional Trauma-Informed Care Coordination (social worker, physician, psychiatrist, nurse, acupuncturist, nutritionist/dietician, occupational therapist, physical therapist, pharmacist, speech therapist, dentist, dental hygienist, educational psychologist, librarian, teacher, case manager):

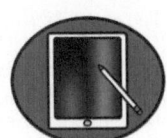

Biological-Psychological-Social
AT Assessment

Please record life challenges, milestones, achievements, past history, current issues, duration, frequency, and onset of symptoms for the developmental themes below. Base the assessment on the themes organized under three domains of functioning: (1) Biological, (2) psychological, and (3) social. These themes are just suggestions for further conversations; they are not exhaustive. AT would suggest close assessment of the important interplay of each of the three domains simultaneously, while dynamically considering the intersection of multiple LGBTQI identities. Reference the Intersectionality Gem worksheet for addition self-assessment data.

Name:	Date of Birth:
Address:	*Reference data from the Intersectionality Gem worksheet*
Phone:	Sex or Assigned Sex at Birth:
Referred by:	Sexual Identity (Orientation):
Emergency Contact: Contact Phone:	Gender Identity:
Insurance/Benefits:	Gender Expression:

Presenting Issue

Interplay

Biological Domain

Age

Health/Wellness Practices

Exercise

Nutrition/Appetite

Sleep Hygiene

Energy/Motivation

Birth Order

Medical Health/History/Diagnosis

Sexual Health/Behavior

Pain/Management

Allergies

Psychopharmacology/Medication Adherence

Substance Abuse/Addictions

Environmental Issues

Toxic Stress/Minority Stress

Physical Abuse/Neglect/Exploitation

LGBTQI Biological Traumas

Medical Family History

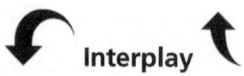 **Interplay**

Psychological Domain

Stress

Mental Health

DSM/ICD Diagnosis

Coping

Thoughts/Cognitions

Suicidal Ideation

Homicidal Ideation

Child/Elder Abuse

Intimate Partner Violence

Mood-Related Issues

Anxiety

Depression

Severe/Persistent Mental Illness

Concentration

Agitation

Bereavement/Loss

Psychological Abuse/Neglect/Exploitation

LGBTQI Psychological Trauma

Motivation for Treatment

Mental Status Exam

Family History of Mental Health

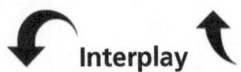 **Interplay**

Social Domains

Cultural/Spiritual Practice

Family (Extended or Choosen Family) History

Children

Friends

School

Work/Career

Church/Temple/Mosque/Organized Religion

Groups/Activity/Interest

Hobbies/Athletics/Leisure/Recreation

Community/Geography

Attachment Figures Growing Up

Relationship Status/History/Goals

Coming Out/Transitions/Identity

Financial Resources/Benefits

Medical Benefits/Insurance

Residential History/Affirming Living Situation

Legal Issues

Incarceration/Arrest

Immigration

Military Service/Veteran/History

Education/History

Employment/History

Loss/Grief

Strengths

LGBTQI Affirming Networks

Referrals/Resources

Biopsychosocial Observations, Non-Pathologizing Differential Diagnosis Formulation (if required), and Interpretive Summary

Appendix C

Resources

WEBSITES

- GLAAD
- The Williams Institute
- Human Rights Campaign (HRC)
- Lambda Legal
- NoH8 Campaign
- Over the Rainbow Book List
- The Trevor Project
- Southerners On New Ground (SOND)
- LGBTQ Parenting Network
- SAGE: Advocating and Services for LGBT Elders
- ILGA World – the International Lesbian, Gay, Bisexual, Trans and Intersex Association
- PLAG
- GSA Network
- GLSEN
- It Gets Better Project
- National Center for Transgender Equality
- The Audre Lorde Project
- Harvey Milk Foundation
- ACT UP
- amfAR, The Foundation for AIDS Research
- Council on Social Work Education (CSWE)
- Victory Fund
- Lesbian Herstory Archives
- Matthew Shepard Foundation
- National LGBTQ Task Force
- Queer Nation NY
- Transgender Law Center
- National Association of Social Workers (NASW)
- Headspace
- Balance
- Mindshift CBT
- Toxic Thinking: Awareness and Prevention

BOOKS

- *The Deviant's War* – by Eric Cervini (Macmillan, 2020)
- *Crip Theory: Cultural Signs of Queerness and Disability* – by Robert McRuer (NYU Press, 2008)
- *The Stonewall Reader* – by Edmund White (Penguin Classics, 2019)

- *Real Queer America: LGBT Stories from Red States* – by Samantha Allen (Black Bay Books, 2020)
- *The Lavender Scare* – by David Johnson (University of Chicago Press, 2006)
- *The Queer and Transgender Resilience Workbook* – by Anneliese Singh (New Harbinger Publications, 2018)
- *Black on Both Sides: A Racial History of Trans Identity* – by C. Riley Snorton (University of Minnesota Press, 2017)
- *LGBTQ Clients in Therapy* – by Joe Kort (Norton, 2018)
- *Trans Allyship Workbook* – by Davey Shlasko (Think Again, 2017)
- *Sister Outsider* – by Audre Lorde (Crossing Press, 2007)
- *Social Work Practice with the LGBTQ Community* – by Michael Dentato (Oxford, 2018)
- *Affirmative Counseling with LGBTQI+ People* – by Misty Ginicola, Cheri Smith, and Joel Filmore (Wiley, 2017)
- *Transgender History: The Roots of Today's Revolution* (2nd ed.) – by Susan Stryker (Seal Press, 2017)
- *Love Wins* – by Debbie Cenziper and Jim Obergefell (William Marrow, 2017)
- *Queer Social Work: Cases for LGBTQ+ Affirmative Practice* – by Tyler Argüello (Columbia University Press, 2019)
- *The Celluloid Closet: Homosexuality in the Movies* – by Vito Russo (Harper and Row, 1987)
- *A Quick Guide to the Cass Theory of Gay and Lesbian Identity Formation* – by Vivienne Cass (Brightfire, 2015)
- *A Guide to Gender: The Social Justice Advocate's Handbook* (2nd ed.) – by Sam Killerman (Impetus Books, 2017)
- *Counseling LGBTI Clients* – by Kevin Alderson (Sage, 2013)
- *Mindfulness and Acceptance for Gender and Sexual Minorities* – by Matthew Skinta, Aisling Curtin, and John Pachankis (New Harbinger Publications, 2016)
- *LGBTQ-Parent Families* (2nd ed.) – by Abbie Goldberg and Katherine Allen (Springer, 2020)
- *Middlesex: A Novel* – by Jeffrey Eugenides (Macmillan, 2002)
- *The Gay Revolution* – by Lillian Faderman (Simon & Schuster, 2015)
- *And the Band Played On* – by Randy Shilts (St. Martin's Press, 2007)
- *How to Survive a Plague* – by David France (Vintage, 2017)
- *When We Rise* – by Cleve Jones (Hachette Books, 2017)
- *The Men with the Pink Triangle* – by Heinz Heger (Alyson Books, 1994)
- *This Day in June* – by Gayle Pitman and Kristyna Litten (Magination Press, 2014)
- *Transgender Warriors: Making History from Joan of Arc to Dennis Rodman* – by Leslie Feinberg (Beacon Press, 1997)
- *The Gender Quest Workbook: A Guide for Teens and Young Adults Exploring Gender Identity* – by Rylan Jay Testa, Deborah Coolhart, and Jayme Peta (Instant Help, 2015)
- *The ABC's of LGBT+* – by Ashley Mardell (Mango Media, 2016)
- *The Art Activity Book for Relational Work* – by Jennifer Guest (Jessica Kingsley, 2017)
- *My New Gender Workbook* – by Kate Bornstein (Routledge, 2013)

NOTES AND REFLECTIONS

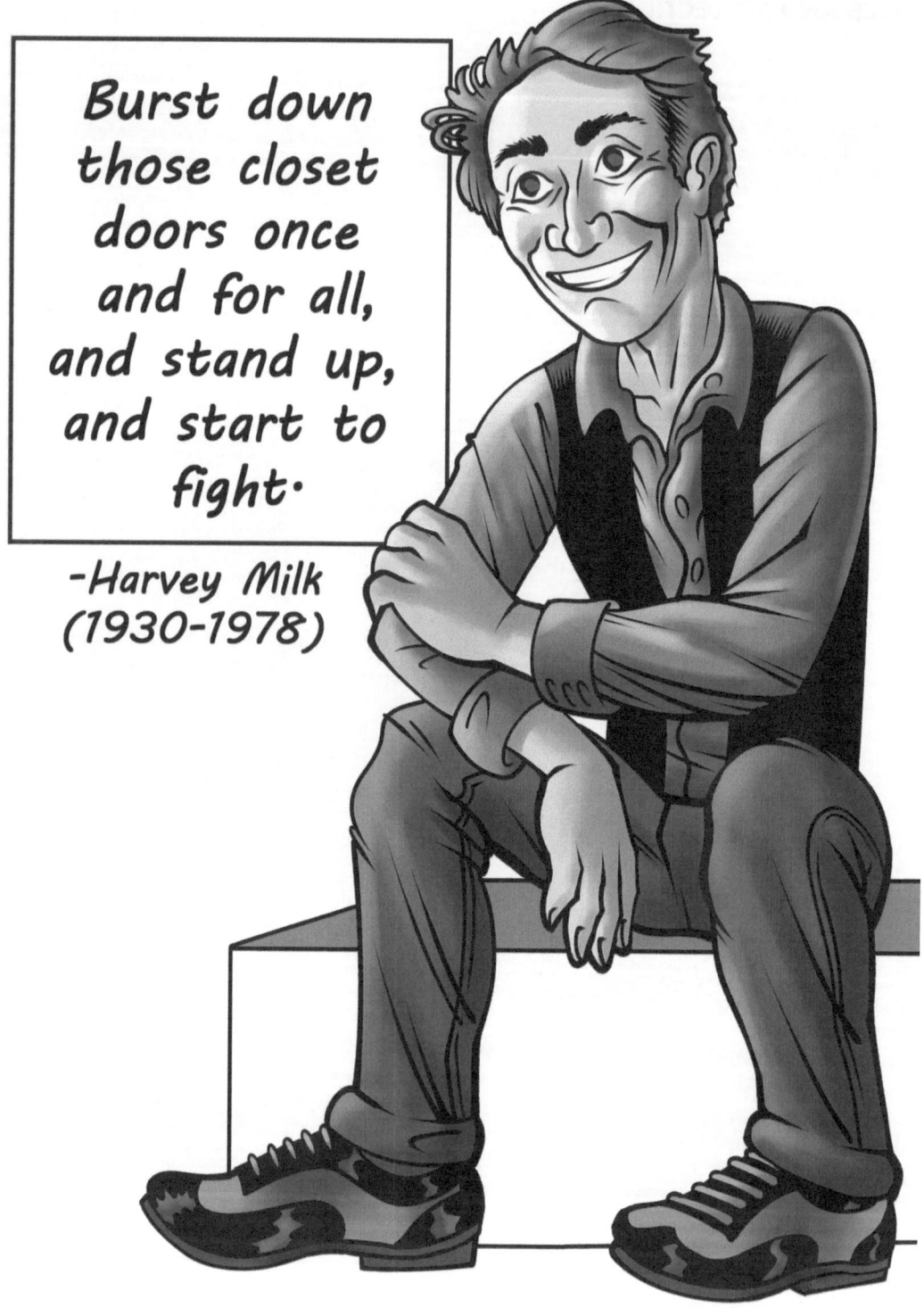

Burst down those closet doors once and for all, and stand up, and start to fight.

-Harvey Milk
(1930-1978)

Future Life Selfie

In the space below place a selfie, doodle, drawing, stickers, stamps, words, or cut-and-paste printed images that represents what you want to continue to feel and think about yourself in the future.

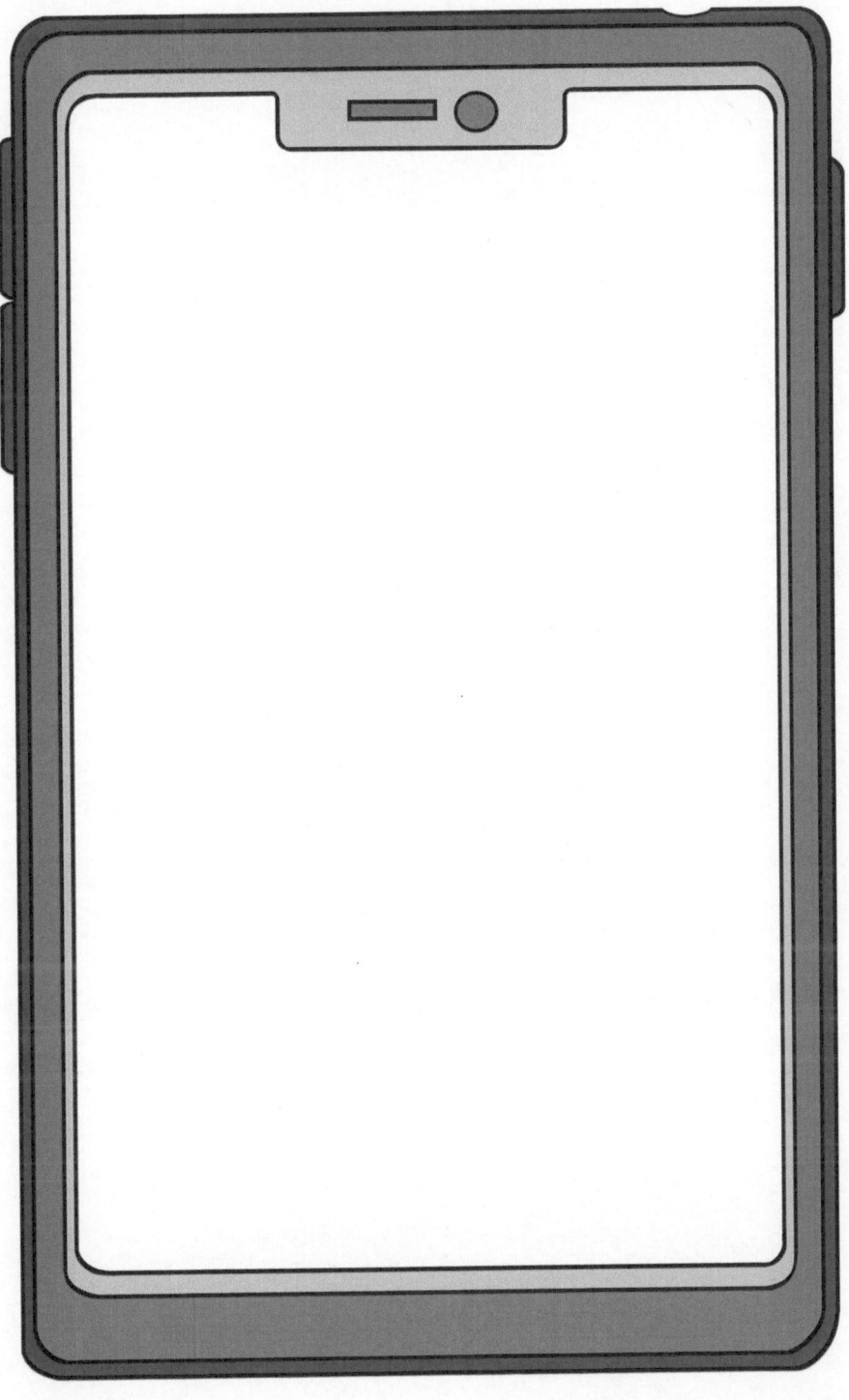

References

Alderson, K. (2013). *Counseling LGBTI clients.* Sage Publications, Inc.

Allison, R. (2012, May). *Ten things transgender persons should discuss with their healthcare provider.* GLMA: Health Professionals Advancing LGBTQ Equality. http://www.glma.org/index.cfm?fuseaction=Page.viewPage&pageID=692

Beck, J. S. (2020). *Cognitive therapy: Basics and beyond* (3rd ed.). The Guilford Press.

Blosnich, J. R., Henderson, E. R., Coulter, R. W. S., Goldbach, J. T., & Meyer, I. H. (2020). Sexual orientation change efforts, adverse childhood experiences, and suicide ideation and attempt among sexual minority adults, United States, 2016–2018. *American Journal of Public Health, 110,* 1024–1030.

Bowlby, J. (1969). *Attachment and loss: Volume 1* (2nd ed.). Basic Books.

Brofenbrenner, U. (1989). Ecological systems theory. In R. Vasta (Ed.), *Annals of child development: Six theories of child development: Revised formulations and current issues* (pp. 187–247). JAI Press.

Burnes, T. R., Dexter, M. M., Richmond, K., Singh, A. A., & Cherrington, A. (2016). The experiences of transgender survivors of trauma who undergo social and medical transition. *Traumatology, 22*(1), 75.

Centers for Disease Control (2016, February 29). *For your health: Recommendations for a healthier you.* https://www.cdc.gov/msmhealth/for-your-health.htm

Conron, K. J., Mimiaga, M. J., & Landers, S. J. (2010). A population-based study of sexual orientation identity and gender differences in adult health. *American Journal of Public Health, 100*(10), 1953–1960.

Crenshaw, K. (1989). Demarginalizing the intersection of race and sex: A black feminist critique of antidiscrimination doctrine, feminist theory and antiracist politics. *University of Chicago Legal Forum,* 140, 139.

DeJong, P., & Berg, I. K. (1998). *Interviewing for solutions.* Brooks.

Dinno, A. (2017). Homicide rates of transgender individuals in the United States: 2010–2014. *American Journal of Public Health, 107*(9), 1441–1447.

Dreeben, S. J., Mamberg, M. H., & Salmon, P. (2013). The MBSR body scan in clinical practice. *Mindfulness, 4*(4), 394–401.

Eubanks-Carter, C., & Goldfried, M. R. (2006). The impact of client sexual orientation and gender on clinical judgments and diagnosis of borderline personality disorder. *Journal of Clinical Psychology, 62*(6), 751–770.

Fitzpatrick, K. (2017, August 1). Why adult coloring books are good for you. *CNN Health.* https://www.cnn.com/2016/01/06/health/adult-coloring-books-popularity-mental-health/index.html

Ginicola, M. M., Smith, C., & Filmore, J. M. (Eds.). (2017). *Affirmative counseling with LGBTQI+ people.* John Wiley & Sons.

Goldbach, J., & Dunlap, S. (2016). Social work practice with sexual minorities. In E. Schott & E. Weiss (Eds.), *Transformative social work practice* (pp. 379–398). Sage Publications, Inc.

Goodrich, K. M., & Ginicola, M. M. (2017). Evidence-based practice for counseling the LGBTQI+ population. In M. M. Ginicola, C. Smith, & J. M. Filmore (Eds.), *Affirmative counseling with LGBTQI+ people.* John Wiley & Sons.

Killerman, S. (2017). *A guide to gender: The social justice advocate's handbook* (2nd ed.). Impetus Books.

Kort, J. (2018). *LGBTQ clients in therapy: Clinical issues and treatment strategies.* W. W. Norton and Company.

Langenderfer-Magruder, L., Walls, N. E., Whitfield, D. L., Brown, S. M., & Barrett, C. M. (2016). Partner violence victimization among lesbian, gay, bisexual, transgender, and queer youth: Associations among risk factors. *Child and Adolescent Social Work Journal, 33*(1), 55–68.

MacLean, P. D. (1990). *The triune brain in evolution: Role in paleocerebral functions.* Springer Science + Business Media.

Maslow, A. H. (1987). *Motivation and personality* (3rd ed.). Pearson Education.

Maylon, A. K. (1982). Psychotherapeutic implications for internalized homophobia in gay men. In J. C. Gonsiorek (Ed.), *Homosexuality and psychotherapy: A practitioner's handbook for affirmative models* (pp. 59–70). Haworth Press.

McKinnish, T. R., Burgess, C., & Sloan, C. A. (2019). Trauma-informed care of sexual and gender minority patients. In M. R. Gerber (Ed.), *Trauma-informed healthcare approaches* (pp. 85–105). Springer.

Mizock, L., & Lewis, T. K. (2008). Trauma in transgender populations: Risk, resilience, and clinical care. *Journal of Emotional Abuse, 8*(3), 335–354.

Pachankis, J. E., Hatzenbuehler, M. L., Rendina, H. J., Safren, S. A., & Parsons, J. T. (2015). LGB-affirmative cognitive-behavioral therapy for young adult gay and bisexual men: A randomized controlled trial of a transdiagnostic minority stress approach. *Journal of Consulting and Clinical Psychology, 83*(5), 875–889. doi: 10.1037/ccp0000037

Pagan, A. (2018, June 6). Power up for pride with LGBTQ+ superheroes! New York Public Library. https://www.nypl.org/blog/2018/06/06/power-pride-lgbtq-superheroes-graphic-novels

Petrecca, L. (2019, March 22). *Dating safety in age of technology.* AARP. https://www.aarp.org/home-family/dating/info-2019/online-dating-safety.html

Poteat, T. (2012, May). *Top 10 things lesbians should discuss with their healthcare provider.* GLMA: Health Professionals Advancing LGBTQ Equality. http://www.glma.org/index.cfm?fuseaction=Page.viewPage&pageID=691

Prochaska, J. O., Redding, C. A., & Evers, K. E. (2015). The transtheoretical model and stages of change. In K. Glanz, B. K. Rimer, & V. Viswanath (Eds.), *Health behavior: Theory, research, and practice* (pp. 125–148). Jossey-Bass.

Richmond, K. A., Burnes, T., & Carroll, K. (2012). Lost in trans-lation: Interpreting systems of trauma for transgender clients. *Traumatology, 18*(1), 45–57.

Richmond, K., Burnes, T. R., Singh, A. A., & Ferrara, M. (2017). *Assessment and treatment of trauma with TGNC clients: A feminist approach.* In A. Singh & l. m. dickey (Eds.), *Affirmative counseling and psychological practice with transgender and gender nonconforming clients* (pp. 191–212). American Psychological Association.

Rosenwohl-Mack, A., Tamar-Mattis, S., Baratz, A. B., Dalke, K. B., Ittelson, A., et al. (2020). A national study on the physical and mental health of intersex adults in the US. *PLOS ONE, 15*(10): e0240088. https://doi.org/10.1371/journal.pone.0240088

Ross, A. (2015, January 26). Berlin story: How the Germans invented gay rights- more than a century ago. *The New Yorker.* https://www.newyorker.com/magazine/2015/01/26/berlin-story

Sanders, C., Carter, B., & Lwin, R. (2015). Young women with a disorder of sex development: Learning to share information with health professionals, friends and intimate partners about bodily differences and infertility. *Journal of Advanced Nursing, 71*(8), 1904–1913.

Savoy, M., O' Gurek, D., & Brown-James, A. (2020). Sexual health history: Techniques and tips. *American Family Physician, 101*(5), 286–293.

Scheer, J. R., Harney, P., Esposito, J., & Woulfe, J. M. (2019). Self-reported mental and physical health symptoms and potentially traumatic events among lesbian, gay, bisexual, transgender, and queer individuals: The role of shame. *Psychology of Violence.* https://doi.apa.org/doiLanding?doi=10.1037%2Fvio0000241

Shapiro, F. (2017). *Eye movement desensitization and reprocessing (EMDR) therapy: Basic principles, protocols, and procedures.* Guilford Publications.

Sudak, D. M., Majeed, M. H., & Youngman, B. (2014). Behavioral activation: A strategy to enhance treatment response. *Journal of Psychiatric Practice, 20*(4), 269–275. doi: 10.1097/01.pra.0000452563.05911.c9

Tambe, M., & Rice, E. (Eds.). (2018). *Artificial intelligence and social work.* Cambridge University Press.

Toren, A. (2018). *HIV: Why see a specialist?* Healthgrades. https://www.healthgrades.com/right-care/hiv/hiv-why-see-a-specialist

Winn, R. (2012, May). *Ten things gay men should discuss with their healthcare provider.* GLMA: Health Professionals Advancing LGBTQ Equality. http://glma.org/index.cfm?fuseaction=Page.viewPage&pageID=690

Index